Austin [illegible]

LOVE HIM ANYWAY

Sara,

We love because he
first loved us.
1 John 4:19

Abby Banks

Wyatt

"*Love Him Anyway* is an incredible story of love, hope, loss, and the strength of a family and more importantly a Mamma on a mission. Abby truly is an inspiration to all, and her writing is real and powerful and truly reminds you that life happens and although things might not go the way we planned, we can't stop living, loving, and trusting in God's plan. I am truly inspired by Wyatt and his amazing Mamma!"

—VICTORIA ARLEN,
ESPN On Air Personality, Paralympic Gold Medalist, and
Transverse Myelitis Survivor

"I highly recommend *Love Him Anyway* to anyone who is dealing with any sort of obstacle in life. Wyatt has had to deal with adversity at a very young age but chooses to be happy and live life to the fullest. His story is a triumph of the human spirit and a reminder that life is worth celebrating even in the hard moments."

—ERIC LEGRAND,
Former Rutgers University Football Player
and Spinal Cord Injury Activist

"Rejoice in the Lord always. Easy to do when your Christian life is going well. But it is an entirely different undertaking when you wake up one morning and life as you knew it the night before no longer exists. Such is the case in this poignant, thoughtfully written story of a tenacious little boy's strength and courage, the love of his mother, and the beautiful tapestry woven in community during trying times. Heartbreaking yet full of hope and resiliency,

Love Him Anyway reminds us all that no suffering is wasted and God uses our most difficult times for His greatest glory."

—HEATHER GRAY BLALOCK,
Author of *Faith, Hope, Love & Deployment*

"*Love Him Anyway* presents a story of love and triumph through the eyes of a mother who has lived an experience that no one can imagine, until it happens to them. Transverse Myelitis struck her youngest son, Wyatt, at the age of 7 months and their lives changed. While terrifying and grim at first glance, Abby Banks is able to tell a story of truth, hope, opportunities, and possibilities of what their family has experienced in this journey and what they look forward to in years to come. With faith and strength and acknowledgment of God as their Higher Power, Abby has created a 'how to' story of Wyatt's story. It is without reservation that OPAF recommends *Love Him Anyway* and with pride that the Banks crew has become part of our family."

—ROBIN BURTON,
Executive Director Orthotic & Prosthetic Activities Foundation
(OPAF) & The First Clinics

"Imagine you are at work or just playing and your arms, legs, and torso start to tingle. You think you're tired and just need to rest. Little do you know that your body is betraying you at that moment and is attacking your spinal cord; in a matter of hours you will be paralyzed. It happened to me, and it happened to Wyatt. *Love Him Anyway* is a powerful story of hardship, determination, and conquest. Have your tissues ready! Let Wyatt's story spur you to spread awareness and support funding for transverse myelitis research."

—MIKE L. JEZDIMIR,
Chairman Mike L. Jezdimir Foundation and Transverse Myelitis Survivor

"The story of *Love Him Anyway* grips the heart in such a personal way because Abby faces one of every mother's fears—watching her child suffer with no way to stop it. But as difficult the experience, and as much as she would want to run away from God, Abby's story is about running toward the God of all hope. Abby encourages the reader to move from a place of brokenness to a place of celebration."

—SARAH BRAGG
Author of *Body. Beauty. Boys. The Truth About Girls and How We See Ourselves* and host Surviving Sarah podcast

LOVE HIM ANYWAY

Finding Hope in the Hardest Places

ABBY BANKS

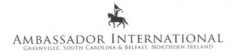

Ambassador International
GREENVILLE, SOUTH CAROLINA & BELFAST, NORTHERN IRELAND

www.ambassador-international.com

Love Him Anyway
Finding Hope in the Hardest Places

ISBN: 978-1-62020-572-3
eISBN: 978-1-62020-596-9

Cover Design and Page Layout by Hannah Nichols
eBook Conversion by Anna Riebe Raats

Photo Page 160: Dani Dunn Photography
Author Photo and Photo Page 218: Palmetto Posh Photography

AMBASSADOR INTERNATIONAL
Emerald House
411 University Ridge, Suite B14
Greenville, SC 29601, USA
www.ambassador-international.com

AMBASSADOR BOOKS
The Mount
2 Woodstock Link
Belfast, BT6 8DD, Northern Ireland, UK
www.ambassadormedia.co.uk

The colophon is a trademark of Ambassador

To Jason
Thank you for loving me anyway

To Jay, Austin, Wyatt
I will always love you anyway and in every way

Even youths grow tired and weary,

And young men stumble and fall;

But those who hope in the Lord will renew their strength.

They will soar on wings like eagles;

They will run and not grow weary,

They will walk and not be faint.

~ Isaiah 40:30–31

CONTENTS

INTRODUCTION

AS A YOUNG ADULT, I embarked on life's journey with specific expectations for the route my family would travel. I had chosen a path marked by beauty, triumph, and dreams come true. It was perfect. It was what I wanted for myself, my husband, and especially for my children.

Then one night, I put my beloved baby boy to bed. He was happy, healthy, and whole. By morning, he was paralyzed. And just like that, we were swept from the pretty path and forced into a strange wilderness of daunting mountains without a map to guide us. I was left wondering whether God had deserted us.

The dramatic destruction of my expectations made my heart ache in ways I never thought possible, and I have struggled to come to terms with our reality. My precious Wyatt is still paralyzed, and I can't understand why God didn't make it all better. I could drown myself in a sea of anger because life hasn't turned out the way I planned, but I know that life is a gift, and I want to fight to make ours amazing, no matter what it looks like.

When sin entered the world, it broke everything. Nothing is as it should be. Marriages end. Children get sick. Addiction takes control. Infertility happens. Parents walk out. Dreams get crushed. The hard happens, and it is no respecter of age, race, religion, or social status. There is brokenness in us all.

My family's battles are easy to see. There is a little boy in an orange chair who rolls beside me. It's unmistakable. Brokenness found us. Your battles might not be so visible. Your scars may be hidden, but all of our hearts bear wounds from our brokenness. I wish I could glue us all back together and keep the hurt out, but I can't. I can only point you to the One who can make you whole.

I wish I had a different story tell, one that was a little easier to live, but this is the story I have been given. My heart longs to make good from the bad, to see purpose come from pain. I want to encourage you to keep fighting in whatever storm you're facing. God is near, my friend, even if you can't feel Him. It is my prayer that my words will remind you of who He is. The route my life has taken is not what I had planned, but the destination is the same. I am certain of it.

God may not have moved my mountain, but He moved me. His hand carried me. It is by His strength alone that I've been able to face each day, and He can do the same for you. I will not mourn the lost expectations. I will celebrate the life that remains. I will celebrate the life I didn't plan, the lessons learned, the milestones achieved, the friendships made, and the community I now belong to. I will look to the top of my mountain with eager anticipation. The climb will be hard, but the summit will be glorious.

CHAPTER 1

SURPRISE, SURPRISE

"For I know the plans I have for you," declares the LORD,
*"plans to prosper you and not to harm you, plans to give you
hope and a future."*

~ Jeremiah 29:11

TWO PINK LINES STARED BACK at me, and it was all I could do to keep myself from passing out in the shower. I didn't know whether to laugh or cry. This was not what I had planned. God's timing seemed humorous and completely amiss. Jason and I had struggled for years with infertility, and the idea that we could get pregnant on our own seemed like a fairy tale reserved for pretty people with perfect lives. We were definitely not that, and our first two children had the glamorous distinction of being conceived in a doctor's office. Jason still takes great joy in my embarrassment when he tells people that there were three people in the room when our first two kids were made. Our oldest, Jay, was five, and our daughter, Austin, was only nine months old when that dollar store test told me I was pregnant with Wyatt.

My heart had longed for a third child. During our infertility treatments, I prayed for multiples. I wanted lots of babies and a minivan full of car seats. We once had to cancel a cycle when my fertility drugs worked a little too well. I had eight eggs, and since we weren't open to selective reduction, we couldn't move forward and had to wait another month before we could try again. Jason was adamant he didn't want to raise a basketball team. I was heartbroken and wanted to try anyway, hoping that we might have twins or triplets. I think all the hormones I was on must have clouded my judgment, and I became inconsolable and irrational. I cried so much after that appointment that Jason actually stopped and bought me a red couch on the way home. I still wonder what the poor salesman must have thought. My eyes were red and still filled with tears, and I'm pretty sure Jason uttered the words, "Just give her whatever she wants."

When we found out we were pregnant for a second time, I crossed my fingers and held my breath, hoping for two heartbeats. It was greedy of me. I know that, but I was secretly disappointed when we saw only one tiny black and white flicker on the screen. Jason was not so secretly relieved. He's much more practical and level-headed than I am. One baby at a time was all he could handle. I wanted more children, but I knew we weren't going to shell out a small fortune a third time for infertility treatments. And honestly, I didn't want to go through the physical and emotional stress of infertility treatments again. I accepted that we would have only two children. I was thankful that God had given me two amazing children, but I held out hope that God would lead us to adoption down the road. I never expected that God would allow me to carry another child myself.

I realize that I should have thrown my hands in the air and yelled, "Thank you, Jesus!" when I saw a positive pregnancy test, but I didn't. I stared at it, shaking my head in disbelief. Instead of celebrating, I was wondering how I could possibly take care of one more person. It was awful and completely selfish, but I was tired. So very tired. I feel guilty now for thinking it, but the months following Austin's birth were so difficult. The good days had been exhausting, and the bad days seemed almost unbearable. I just didn't know how much more I could handle.

Austin's birth did not go as planned. She and I were both healthy, but everything else went terribly wrong. Family members were missing, and while Jason was thrilled for the birth of his daughter, his heart was breaking into pieces. His mom, who was already suffering from Alzheimer's, was diagnosed with a large bowel obstruction and a life-threatening infection the day Austin was born. She needed emergency surgery; all indications were that she had a large, cancerous mass in her stomach. We weren't given much hope. Jason and the rest of his family gathered in a hospital an hour away from me, praying that she would survive surgery. I sat alone in an empty hospital room nursing my newborn while waiting for an update. Minutes seemed like hours, and hours seemed like days as I listened to excited visitors shuffling in and out of neighboring rooms. The quiet of my room was broken only by the cries of my precious new daughter until the phone finally rang. Jason's mom had survived surgery, but she needed a colostomy to save her life. Two days later, we got the news. There was no cancer. Praise God! We felt so much relief.

Despite the good news, Jason's mom was still very sick, and it was too much for his dad to handle on his own. Jason and I quickly put all our belongings in storage and moved into his parents' house to help care for her. I shed many tears as we wrapped china in bubble wrap and boxed away years of memories. It was tough and humbling for me, and I realized that this is what God meant when He said, "Honor your father and mother." It was not what I wanted to do, but I knew it was what we were supposed to do.

Jason's mom came home from the hospital after a month-long stay with a PICC line and IV medications. She needed five infusions a day that each took nearly two hours to run completely. A rehab nurse gave me a quick crash course on how to administer them, and I became a nurse overnight. Middle of the night baby feedings doubled as IV hook-up times. It was exhausting, but the IV medications seemed like a day at the beach compared to teaching someone with Alzheimer's how to care for a colostomy.

There were lots of accidents. Lots of smells. Lots of poop. Lots of middle of the night tears. Lots of self-pity. Lots of "why me?" I will spare you all the intricate details, but it was awful. Between baby diapers and colostomy bags, I felt like I was living in a Porta-John at a summer festival. Life was pretty crappy, literally and figuratively. By the grace of God, we all survived, and soon Jason's entire family were experts at colostomy bag care. We felt like we had defeated the dragon, like we had been put through the fire and came out stronger.

Then Jason got sick.

He tried to be manly and tough it out, but I forced him to go see a doctor. I actually went with him to make sure he conveyed the seriousness of the situation to his doctor. He had been in so much pain, and I knew something was wrong. His doctor listened and immediately sent him to the hospital for a CT scan. Who would believe that almost nine months to the day of his mom's surgery, Jason would face the same fate? A nurse came into the waiting room with Jason's family doctor on the phone. I didn't need to hear the conversation. The tears that rolled down Jason's face told me all I needed to know. His bowel had perforated, and he needed emergency surgery.

We were immediately sent over to the emergency room, where Jason was assessed and the surgery team was called back to the hospital since it was now well after 6 pm. It all happened so quickly. We called all our friends and family to let them know what had transpired. We held hands. We cried. And we prayed. I think we were in shock. Jason kept apologizing to me like he had done something to cause this to happen. I just kept telling him how much I loved him, and we joked about living out "in sickness and in health."

When the surgeon finally arrived, he came into the ER to explain the surgery. He said that he would locate the perforation, cut out the bad portion, and clean up the area. He explained that if there wasn't too much infection, he would reconnect Jason's bowels. Then he proceeded to say that there was probably too much damage for that option and started explaining to us what a colostomy was. I quit listening. I didn't need an explanation. I knew all too well what was about to happen, and I began praying that the doctor was wrong.

Jason's dad and my parents arrived just before Jason was taken back into surgery. We all prayed together in the ER before the surgery team came to take Jason away. I kissed him one last time and assured him that everything was going to be okay. Jason's dad, my parents, and I were all led into a dark hallway. Since all the normal waiting rooms had already closed up, they had to find somewhere for us to wait. We ended up in a pre-op assessment room. All the rooms around us were dark and empty—much like the sentiments of my own heart during those anxious moments.

I didn't say much while we waited. The others tried to keep the mood light, but my heart was heavy. I walked the dark hallway and prayed. I wasn't praying for survival. I knew he would make it through surgery without any problems, but my heart ached at the thought of him waking up with a colostomy. I didn't want that for him, and I knew how badly he didn't want it. So I prayed. I walked. I waited. I hoped.

The surgery was taking longer than expected, and just as my nerves were getting the best of me, a nurse popped her head into the room, and said that Jason had done great and was in recovery. She told me the doctor would be out soon, but I could go back and be with Jason until the doctor was ready to talk with us. I wasn't brave enough to ask if he had needed a colostomy. I didn't want to hear the answer. So I just followed the nurse through the maze of hallways to the recovery room.

It was a huge room, and Jason was resting by himself in the corner alone. I kissed his forehead and grabbed his hand. As I looked down, my heart sank. There *it* was, lying next to his leg on the bed. A box of colostomy bags. No questions needed to be asked. I knew what had happened.

I was devastated, but Jason handled it like a champion. He felt lucky to be alive and never once complained. His recovery wasn't easy. It was painful and uncomfortable in so many ways. The man who never liked to ask for help, needed it so much, but in typical Jason fashion, he laughed his way through it all. We found comfort in reminding each other that it could have been worse, and we were overjoyed when the doctor told us Jason's colostomy could be reversed after three to four months of healing.

I started feeling sick a few days after Jason's surgery. I was even more tired than usual, and I thought I had a stomach virus. I blamed it on stress, hospital germs, and sleeping in a recliner, but it didn't go away. Jason was in the hospital for ten days, and the morning after I brought him home, I decided to take an old pregnancy test, thinking there was no way it could possibly be positive. I took the test before I hopped in the shower and sat it on the side of the bathtub. I was almost done with my shower when I remembered that I hadn't looked back at the test. I reached down, and as I brought it closer, my heart seemed to skip a beat. Really? I couldn't believe my own eyes. There were two dark pink lines. There was no question that it was positive, and I was overwhelmed. We were having a third child.

I woke Jason up from a drug-induced sleep to tell him the news. He was still doped-up on pain medication, and he had trouble following my broken words. I sat on the edge of the bed and started talking before he even had a chance to open his eyes. I was crying and blabbering like a crazy lady. I remember saying that I didn't know how it happened, and I apologized for the bad timing. He finally cut me off and asked if I was pregnant. When I said yes, he just grabbed me and held me close.

"That's wonderful," he said as he squeezed me tightly in his arms.

Instantly, all my fears were erased, and I thanked God for the child growing inside me.

After my initial selfish thoughts, I saw Wyatt as a gift from God. He was my reward for surviving the previous nine months, and I praised God every time I felt that sweet baby move. He was a miracle, and although I didn't believe it at first, he was right on time. I felt like the sun was shining on my face again, and I enjoyed every minute of it. My pregnancy was a breeze, and Jason and I both breathed a big, simultaneous sigh of relief when our ultrasounds revealed we were having a healthy boy. We never took for granted that our children would be born healthy, and we held our breath waiting for the comforting "Everything looks perfect!" during all our children's first ultrasounds.

Life returned to a normal rhythm, and it was like a balm to my weary soul. Before I knew it, Jason had healed and was ready for his colostomy reversal. It was the end of a bad dream for him, but for me, it was a finish line. I was ready for the season of suffering to be over, and his surgery signaled the start of a new spring in my heart. He was healthy. His mom grew stronger. We were able to move back into our own home, and I was ready for my surprise miracle baby to be born.

The last few weeks of pregnancy are torture for every woman, and I was no different. My due date was circled on the calendar, and the days were crossed off like a child waiting for the first day of summer vacation. The excitement in my heart grew as the days clicked away, but sorrow found my family for a third time surrounding the births of my children. Two weeks after the birth of Jay, my grandfather passed away, and shortly after Austin was born, my grandmother joined my grandfather in heaven. I hated that my mom wasn't able to celebrate her new grandchildren without mourning a great loss. I had hoped that the birth of Wyatt would be different, but it was not to be.

The Lord gives, and the Lord takes away. And two weeks before Wyatt's birth, He took away again. My aunt died suddenly, without warning. We are but a breath, and tomorrow is not promised. Attending a funeral with a very pregnant belly reminds you how fleeting and temporal this life really is. I hated that my mom had to be faced with that reality yet again, and I hoped that Wyatt's birth would be the medicine that her broken heart needed. She needed something to celebrate. We all needed something to celebrate.

I was completely spoiled during my first two deliveries. Completely, utterly spoiled, and I'm happy to admit it. I'll never forget the words of my doctor during my delivery with Jay. I had just sent the anesthesiologist away because I didn't think it was time for an epidural since I wasn't hurting yet.

"Abby," my doctor said, "this world is full of pain that I can't stop, but I can stop you from hurting during labor. Now, I'm going to send the anesthesiologist back in here. He's going to ask if you want an epidural and you're going to say yes. Quit trying to be tough."

"Yes, sir," I said quickly.

The anesthesiologist came back in, and I never felt a single contraction. I napped, did office work, and talked with my family all day. No pain. No crying. No crazy Lamaze-style breathing. It was the stuff pregnancy dreams are made of, and I was lucky enough to have it happen twice. I scheduled Wyatt's inductions for September 26, 2012, assuming I would have another dream labor.

Jason likes to tell me that one should never assume anything. I assumed, and I was wrong. Wyatt would not wait. As I was lying down for bed one night, I felt a stomach cramp. I got up to watch television to keep from waking Jason with my tossing and turning. Somewhere in the middle of changing channels, I realized I was having more cramps at regular intervals. I finally realized that these cramps might actually be contractions. This was my first "real" labor, and it took me way longer to catch on than it should have. Since I wasn't completely sure, I downloaded a "contraction timer" app on my phone and counted contractions throughout the night. (Yes, there really is an app for that!) By 4 am, my contractions were five minutes apart, and I was pretty uncomfortable. I called my doctor's office and was told it was time to head to the hospital.

I woke Jason up and let him know I was in labor and it was time to go to the hospital. He asked if he had time to take a shower. I thought he was kidding. He wasn't, and I paced around while he showered. Since Austin and Jay were induced, Jason felt cheated out of racing me to the hospital. He was almost giddy as we got in the car. As I buckled up, I had a strong contraction and grimaced in pain.

"If we get pulled over, make that face again and be a little louder," he said.

I reminded myself how much I loved him and nodded my head.

Things started moving pretty quickly once we got to the hospital. I was still expecting an all-day event and told my parents that there was no need to rush to the hospital. I was wrong again. Less than an hour after I got my epidural, Wyatt was born. He was 7 lbs. 10 oz. of pure perfection. None of our family had arrived at the hospital, and we had plenty of time to soak up those first precious moments with Wyatt alone. It was magical. Jason held Wyatt first, and my heart melted as I watched my husband softly rock our son and whisper into his ear. This was love.

Jason put Wyatt in my arms, and for the third time, I stared into a set of newborn blue eyes and marveled at the handiwork of our Creator. I felt so unworthy. He was not a reward for suffering through hard times. Wyatt was an undeserved gift, straight from the hand of God, and I was blessed to be his mom. He was no accident or surprise. I knew God had a plan and purpose for his life, and I was amazed that I got to be part of it. I held Wyatt close and prayed over the life he would lead. His life was meant to honor God, and I prayed God would give me the strength and courage I needed to instill that truth in him no matter the circumstance.

CHAPTER 2

LIFE INTERRUPTED

God is our refuge and strength, an ever-present help in trouble.

~ Psalm 46:1

I FEEL LIKE I CAN remember every second about the first few months of Jay and Austin's lives. I remember putting Jay in a sweet baby blue onesie with little cars on it and pulling a matching knit hat over his tiny bald head before I buckled him in his car seat for our first trip home. He looked like a toy in the giant seat. I remember being mesmerized by his icy blue eyes. I remember sitting his bouncy seat in the sunlight that was streaming through our back window while hoping and praying that his jaundice would go away. I remember being completely terrified and afraid that we broke our brand new baby after he randomly spit up blood after his first bath, and I remember sitting up all night scared to close my eyes for fear that he would do it again.

I can remember every detail of Austin's squishy newborn face. She had the biggest most squeezable cheeks you've ever seen. They were so big that if you held her at the right angle, her cheeks would hang below her jaw line. I remember dressing her in every shade of pink available and adorning her bald little head with the biggest bows I could find. I remember waking up every three hours for the first six months of her life to satisfy her unquenchable appetite, and I remember a scary fall down the stairs that left me with a pinched nerve and an immense sense of guilt because I dropped my baby. Luckily, my cushy baby girl bounced and was left unfazed and unhurt.

My memories of Wyatt's newborn days aren't so clear. I can look through pictures and tell you about each one, but when I just sit down to tell you about his life before he got sick and everything changed, it all gets blurry. Maybe I was just too tired from chasing after his big brother and sister to catalog each memory. Maybe I spent too much time taking pictures instead of living in the moment. Or maybe my memory is just trying to protect me from the heartache of broken dreams for my precious baby. Maybe that blurriness is simply a storm of past tears protecting me from millions of "what could have beens" that pop into our heads.

Despite the fog in my mind, I know that Wyatt has always been the most content child I've ever seen. From the moment we brought him home and placed him in his sister's pink bassinet, he's just seemed so settled. He's never been demanding. I think there were times he just took a nap because *I* looked tired. I don't even remember waking in the night to feed him. I know I did, but I can't remember it.

I do, however, remember being covered in spit-up. Wyatt spit up everywhere, on everyone, all of the time, just like his big brother had done. We were always armed with what seemed like nine million burp cloths to prepare for his impending eruptions, and we gave fair warning to anyone who wanted to hold him. If you held him, he would spit up on you. It was that simple, but Wyatt's smile was so sweet that most people considered it an even trade. His doctor called him a "happy spitter" because he never got upset, but his reflux left him underweight and looking much different as a newborn than Jay and Austin had.

I have to admit that I was a sucker for a trendy baby product, and I had a handful of pacifiers with little animals sewn onto them for Wyatt. I'm pretty sure I even spent $25 for one with a longhorn bull sewn to it only to have Jay's new Christmas puppy bite through the nipple. It really didn't matter because Wyatt wouldn't take it anyway. He preferred sucking on two fingers, never his thumb. I guess he's always liked to do things a little different from the rest of the world. His Pop affectionately gave him the nickname "Wyatt Two-Finger."

I know those first few months were tough. Three kids are hard. They really are, especially when the youngest two are only seventeen months apart. People will tell you that going from two to three kids isn't that hard, but they're lying. Injecting a third child into a family leaves the parents outnumbered and instantly infuses a little chaos. Jason and I felt like there wasn't quite enough of us to go around, and often we felt like we were succeeding if only one of our three was crying.

It was crazy, but it was worth it. Snuggling with my three munchkins for just five minutes made every sleepless night worth it. Take heart, new mom of three kids, it gets easier. I promise. If Jason and I can make it all work, anyone can.

Somewhere in the midst of all the spit-up, diapers, homework, and dirty clothes, we figured it out. Or maybe the kids just got a little older and it was easier. Either way, we felt confident, and life seemed to be under control—at least, that was our illusion.

Then I saw the lump.

It was the end of April 2013, and I was rushing to finish getting ready before I woke the kids up for school. I dried my hair and brushed my teeth before I grabbed a quick sip of water. In the mirror, I saw a lump move in my throat as I swallowed. It looked like an Adam's apple. I thought I was seeing things. I took another sip of water, but I saw it again and again as I continued to take sips of water. I don't know where I thought the lump was going, but I continued to drink water and watch the lump move to reassure myself that I wasn't crazy.

Jason was still lying in bed waiting for me to finish in the bathroom. I walked into our bedroom, turned the light on, and asked Jason to watch my throat as I drank some water. I asked him if the lump had always been there.

"No," he said. "I promise I would have noticed that on our first date. What is it?"

"Well, I either have thyroid cancer or I'm turning into a man," I joked. "Either way, I guess I need to make a doctor's appointment."

Jason didn't think my joke was very funny. I'm not sure why I immediately knew the lump was on my thyroid, but I never really thought anything different.

I started getting the kids up and ready for school, thinking I'd make an appointment for the doctor in a few days, but my cancer joke scared Jason. He made me call the doctor right away. So just a few hours after I saw the lump in the mirror, Jason and I were sitting in a doctor's office, waiting to get my throat checked out. We make a habit of accompanying each other to any appointments that might result in bad news.

My doctor asked a few standard questions. Jason chimed in with all the information he felt was important, amazingly similar to me filling his doctor's ears with every detail I sensed was pertinent when he was sick. My doctor felt my neck. The lump was hard to miss. He felt it too. He tried to reassure me that most of these lumps are nothing, but he wanted to get it checked out to be sure. Miraculously, he got me in to have an ultrasound the same day. If you've ever waited and worried for weeks for a test, you'll know how ecstatic we were. Jason and I aren't good at waiting for answers to medical questions. Honestly, we're really not very good at waiting for anything.

Jason and I quickly headed across town and found ourselves in an all too familiar situation. Waiting for a test.

"No one is supposed to get sick this year," Jason told me. "We had enough last year."

"I know, I know," I said with a chuckle. "But it's my turn to get sick. I get to take a nap and take a few days off if something is wrong. Plus, if it's cancer, I think thyroid cancer is the good cancer to get."

"That's not funny," Jason said. "It's not cancer."

"I know. It's not going to be cancer—but if it is, I'll be okay," I said.

I left Jason in the waiting area when they called me back for the ultrasound. My ultrasound tech explained what she would be doing and asked me to lie down on the table. I told her that it was as close to a spa as I get so I was going to enjoy lying in a dark, quiet room for a few minutes. I'm pretty sure she thought I had lost my mind.

Once on the table, I positioned myself so that I could see the screen. I've had absolutely no medical training, but I've had lots of experience that makes me an expert in my own mind. I had more ultrasounds than I could possibly could count when we were trying to get pregnant with Jay. Polycystic ovaries taught me that cysts are big black circles on ultrasounds. Fluid filled cysts look like empty circles, and that's what I was hoping to see.

The technician tucked a white piece of paper in my collar to protect my shirt and squirted warm gel onto the front of my neck. She took the ultrasound wand (which I've since learned is called a transducer) and pressed it against my neck. She moved it across my neck as she closely watched the monitor. I'm sure I was talking about something, but all I remember doing was watching the screen. I was waiting for her to stop, waiting for her to stop and measure. And she did. One little cross mark and then another, to measure the distance between them. It wasn't a black empty circle. I didn't know much, but I was sure this wasn't a cyst.

When we finished the ultrasound, the tech told me that the information would be sent to the radiologist, and my doctor would probably have the results in a couple days. As we walked to the car, I told Jason that it didn't look like a cyst, but we'd know in a few days. I'm not sure if he believed my medical expertise or not, but it was enough to keep him worried. I, on the other hand, figured he would worry enough for the both of us, so I didn't need to worry too.

Jason and I took the kids to watch Jay play soccer that same evening. In the middle of cheering Jay on, my doctor called. One of the benefits of living in a small town and having your doctor's wife as your son's teacher is getting quick answers. He said he saw the ultrasound results, and there was definitely a nodule on my thyroid. I needed a biopsy. He would refer me to an ENT. The doctor again tried to reassure me that most of the time these nodules are benign.

I told Jason the news. We decided to wait until after the biopsy to tell our families. There was no point in getting everyone all upset for no reason. A few days later, we strolled into the ENT's office, hoping I could get a biopsy the same day. Wishful thinking. Apparently that doesn't happen.

My ENT told me the biopsy would need to happen at the hospital, but I did have the pleasure of having a giant camera shoved up my nose to look down my throat. Numbing spray is a gift from God. My ENT scheduled the biopsy for the next week, but he told me that even if the results were benign, I would need to have my thyroid removed.

Since surgery was inevitable, we figured it was best to go ahead and tell our families. I really wasn't overly concerned, but I did spend more time online than I should've, searching *thyroid cancer* and *thyroid removal*.

I had to bring a copy of the original ultrasound to my biopsy. So for several days I stared at my ultrasound and compared it to images of "cancerous thyroid ultrasounds." It's not a practice I recommend, but researching gave me the illusion of control in a situation where I had none. I prepared myself for every possible scenario. I knew each type of thyroid cancer and treatment. I knew that I would be fine as long as the doctor didn't tell me that I had anaplastic thyroid cancer. My in-depth online searches taught me that it was incurable, but the odds of having it were slim.

I also spent way too much time reading up on thyroid biopsies. I've never been scared of needles, but the size of the biopsy needle that was going to be put in my neck made me a little queasy and extremely nervous. Jason reassured me that everything would be okay. He went with me the day of the biopsy and tried to keep me laughing while we waited. He's always been able to make stressful situations bearable with his uncanny ability to make people laugh when they want to cry.

I think I was laughing as I left him in the waiting room and walked to the room for my biopsy. There were more people in the room than I expected, and the needle was bigger. Much bigger. It looked like something out of a bad dream or a crazy horror movie. I lay in a chair, listening to the doctor explain the procedure. He explained that the needle would be guided by an ultrasound to make sure it went to the right location. I really didn't care about any of that. I just wanted to know what they were going to put on my neck to make it numb. I can handle pain, but if there is an option to avoid it, I'm going to be first in line to take it.

Thankfully, whatever they used to numb my neck worked. It was uncomfortable but definitely not painful. I left the hospital with a small piece of gauze taped to my neck and a hopeful heart since the lump in my neck now felt much smaller. The biopsy results wouldn't be back until the following week, and I knew I needed to stay busy to keep my mind from worry. I even asked God to keep me from obsessing over the results.

God answered, but not exactly in the way I was expecting.

A few days after my biopsy, as I was getting Austin out of the bath, I noticed a bulge in her stomach just above her groin. I dried her off and lifted her onto the changing table. I gently pushed on her stomach, and the bulge squished back in. My heart sank, and I thought, *Are you serious, God?*

She had a hernia. I was sure of it.

Jason's mom had lots of complications following her surgery, which included several hernias in her abdominal wall. Part of her daily care involved checking to make sure that none of her hernias had strangulated. I was all too familiar with that squishing feeling. I picked up the phone and immediately called Jason.

"So, Austin has a hernia, and I'm going to call the doctor tomorrow. I think she'll need surgery, and I wonder if I can get it done before I have mine," I quickly spouted out.

"What? Are you serious? I'll be home in a minute," he said.

When he walked in the door, he was shaking his head. We seriously laughed about the craziness of it all. We knew hernia surgery on a two-year-old wasn't serious at all, but the timing just made everything seem a little chaotic. I was at the pediatrician's office the next day explaining what had happened. Luckily, he didn't think I was crazy and quickly got me a referral to a pediatric surgeon, even though he didn't feel the hernia himself.

Austin's suspected hernia gave me something else to think about, but it didn't keep me from calling my doctor's office daily to get the results of my biopsy. My appointment was scheduled for a Tuesday morning. On Monday afternoon, the receptionist kindly told me that my results were finally back, but biopsy results must be delivered in person.

I didn't sleep much the night before the appointment. My brain ran through a million scenarios. I was scared. I think I was more worried about how I could take care of everything and everyone than I was about my health. I prayed a lot. It was really one, big long rambling prayer. I asked God to make it nothing. I told Him how hard it would be to have cancer, like He didn't already know. I told Him that I was worried about Jason and the kids. I went on and on about everything that scared me until I realized the one thing my babbling prayer focused on. My comfort.

I was focused on what was easiest for me. I wanted what was most comfortable and convenient, and I was lying in bed telling the Creator of the Universe what I needed. I guess I thought I knew better. Staring at the ceiling, I realize that this wasn't about me.

"Dear God," I prayed, "I really, really don't want cancer. You know that. I don't have to tell You, but I want to honor You more than anything else. If cancer is Your plan, help me honor You through it. Help me bring glory to Your name and give me the strength to bear whatever is ahead."

I closed my eyes and finally drifted off to sleep with the feeling that my biopsy results would not be what we had hoped, but I went to sleep with a settled spirit knowing that God was in control.

The next morning after dropping the kids off at school, Jason and I enjoyed breakfast at Cracker Barrel. Comfort food had become a bit of a tradition for us while waiting for potentially bad medical test results. It started while we were still dating and Jason had a multiple sclerosis scare. Our food tradition hasn't been the best thing for our waistline, but it has definitely been good for our souls. The simple act of eating together and celebrating life as it is, has always been refreshing when our hearts were particularly worried and weary.

After breakfast, Jason held my hand as we walked into the doctor's office. We were taken back to a room where Jason again tried to keep the mood light by making me laugh, but we'd both get quiet whenever footsteps from the outside came close to the door. When the door finally opened, my doctor delivered the news without any hesitation.

"I have your biopsy results," he said. "It is a malignant growth. It is papillary carcinoma, and we'll have to remove your entire thyroid."

Jason's hand reached up and rubbed my shoulder as my doctor began to explain how thyroid cancer was treated. I had researched so much beforehand that I was pretty calm. I knew papillary carcinoma was completely treatable, and I also knew that I wouldn't need any chemotherapy.

Thyroid cancer is treated with radioactive iodine. I would have to go on a special diet for several weeks that removed all iodine from my diet, and then be given radioactive iodine that actually seeks out and kills any remaining thyroid tissue. The only downside was that I would actually have to be quarantined after taking the medicine until all the radioactive material left my body. It was especially dangerous to be around babies and small children.

I wasn't looking forward to being radioactive, but I knew it was better than chemotherapy so I wasn't about to complain. Jason and I sat silently and listened to the doctor finish explaining the surgery to us before we were ushered to another part of the office to officially schedule the surgery.

We sat in the familiar cloth-covered wooden office chairs surrounded by stacks of old magazines as we waited to be called into the scheduling office. It was an experience we had become all too familiar with in our young lives. As I looked at Jason, I saw the first tears roll down his face. He wanted to be strong for me, but it was just too much to hold in. Weeks of worry finally escaped in those tears. He wiped his tears away and quietly whispered, "I'm sorry."

The scheduling office called my name. We scheduled the surgery for two weeks later and left the doctor's talking about how we were going to prepare for everything. As soon as I got into the car, my phone began to ring. I scrambled to find it in the bottom of my purse, and as I pulled it out, I clearly saw the incoming call was my dad. I quickly answered, and for the first time since hearing the diagnosis, I cried as I told him the news. Uttering the words, "I have cancer" to my dad made the reality of my diagnosis finally sink in.

Just a few days later, we were getting ready to take Austin to a consultation with a surgeon. I'd picked her clothes out the night before so I wouldn't have to rush in the morning. I hung the pink hanger with my favorite outfit on her closet doorknob. I dressed her in the cutest little black and white gingham outfit with a white kitty cat appliqué and pants with big ruffles on the bottoms, and I attached a big black bow to a headband and placed it on her head since she still didn't have any hair to hold it. I searched through her drawers and found her laciest white socks. I decided that shoes with squeakers were probably inappropriate for a doctor's office, so I picked out her black patent leather Mary-Janes and buckled them on her sweet, wiggly feet.

"Why did you get her so dressed up to go to a doctor's appointment?" Jason asked.

"I know this surgery isn't going to be a big deal, but in case something goes incredibly wrong, I want the doctor to remember this super cute, little girl so he'll work extra hard to save her," I said.

"You're crazy," Jason said. "But with the way our luck has been running, it makes sense."

We all held hands as we walked from the car to the doctor's office. Austin held tightly onto each of our hands as she counted and waited for us to swing her into the air on three. She threw her little bald head back as she sailed through the air, laughing without a care in the world. As we walked to the door, Jason and I glanced at the adjoining doctor's office.

"Pediatric Neurosurgery," I read aloud. "I know this is inconvenient and the timing is not good, but it could be so much worse. I'm just so thankful we aren't walking through those doors."

"Me too. This is nothing," Jason said.

Austin bounced through the door of the doctor's office, and we sat waiting for the doctor with a sense of relief after being reminded Austin's little surgery was nothing compared to what other kids were facing.

The doctor was great and incredibly kind. Her hernia was not out when the doctor examined her, but as I explained the familiar squish, he said that she likely had an inguinal hernia and would definitely need surgery to repair.

I knew that this wasn't an urgent surgery, and it would probably take quite a while to be scheduled, but I wanted it done. I didn't know what the timeline for my recovery following surgery would be, and I didn't want to have to try to take care of myself and Austin at the same time. I explained the situation to the doctor, and he was able to quickly schedule the surgery for the following week.

Austin's surgery was a simple outpatient procedure. She was scheduled early in the morning since it's always hard to keep little ones happy when they can't eat. We arrived with her favorite pillow and blanket in hand and were quickly taken back to a pre-op room where we dressed her in a little purple hospital gown. She laughed and played and bounced across the hospital bed. She was soaking in the one-on-one attention that she was getting from Mommy and Daddy, completely oblivious to the surgery ahead of her.

Jason and I handed her off to the nurses and waved good-bye as we watched her be carried into the operating room. We returned to the waiting room where we sat with Jason's dad and my parents. I couldn't help but worry whether I had been correct about her hernia. None of her doctors had actually felt the hernia squish back and trusted my account. I was worried that I had put her through an unnecessary surgery.

A short time later, the doctor called Jason and me into the counseling room. The surgery was over, and Austin had done great. The doctor said she did indeed have two hernias that needed to be repaired. He told us they would call us back shortly to be with Austin in recovery, but first there was a nurse who wanted to speak with me. A nurse in scrubs entered the room and introduced herself.

"I was helping in your daughter's surgery and heard that you have thyroid cancer. I just wanted to introduce myself and let you know that everything is going to be okay," she said. "I was diagnosed with thyroid cancer and just went through my radioactive iodine treatment. I'd like to give you my phone number in case you have any questions later."

I couldn't help but marvel at how God had orchestrated everything to provide comfort for me during Austin's surgery. We stood in the room talking for a short time when another nurse entered the room and told us we were needed in recovery immediately. Austin was fine, but she wasn't waking up from surgery well.

We have been told that some kids wake up from anesthesia gently, and others wake up violent and angry. Austin was the latter. She was crying and flailing her arms and legs in the air and trying to pull off all the cords that were attached. I tried to comfort her, but there was nothing I could do to calm her down. Jason ended up pinning her legs between his knees and holding her arms back as he rocked her until she finally calmed down. I think exhaustion finally set in for her.

After a short time, we were headed home. Austin was perfect. You would have never known that she had surgery. Our biggest problem was trying to keep her from doing too much. She wanted to run and jump and climb as soon as we got through the door. We were happy that her surgery was simple and behind us so that we could prepare for my surgery and recovery.

We lined up childcare for the kids and made all the necessary preparations for surgery. I told Jason that I was looking forward to taking lots of naps during my recovery. The weekend before the surgery, I came down with an awful stomach virus. I spent the weekend lying on the bathroom floor. I remember lying on the floor thanking God that I didn't have to go through chemotherapy because I couldn't image feeling like that on a regular basis.

Jason's sister, Mandie, arrived at our house early on the Tuesday morning of my surgery so that I wouldn't have to wake the kids. I peeked in each child's room and gave them a kiss on the head before we left. I wanted to tell them I loved them one last time just in case something terribly unexpected happened. Looking back, I wish I had awakened Wyatt. I wish I had scooped him up in my arms and snuggled him close and tickled his little toes. It would have been the last time he would have ever felt my touch on his legs, feet, or stomach. Instead, I just leaned over the side of his white crib and kissed his head.

My parents met Jason and me at the hospital. They waited with us in the pre-op room. I think they were more nervous than I was. My mom was pulling small gifts and surprises from her giant handbag. Gifts are her love language. I know she wanted her gifts to take my mind off the surgery ahead, but I wasn't really scared. I'd read enough that I was no longer worried about the cancer. I was just worried about waking up with a drain coming out of my neck.

We all said a small prayer together, and I was wheeled off to surgery. I don't remember anything until waking up in my room after surgery. Everything went perfectly, and the cancer was contained within my thyroid. Jason heaved a big sigh of relief, and I took the opportunity to rest. Jason and I both have a habit of saying no to pain medicine, but I decided that I would say yes every time it was offered. There wasn't any reason to hurt if I didn't have to, and I knew that I wouldn't be able to take anything once I got home to the kids.

I slept soundly that night and woke up ready to go home. Jason woke up stiff and tired. Hospital chairs do not make for quality sleep. I had hoped we could go home before lunch time, but an early morning blood test revealed that my potassium was too low. I had to stay until the afternoon to ensure that all my levels returned to normal. We spent the day resting and watching television.

The drain coming out of my neck didn't hurt bad, but it looked scary. I knew it would terrify the kids, but I was terrified of seven-month-old Wyatt trying to grab it. He had a habit of pulling on everything. I had given up wearing dangly earrings and necklaces months ago because they didn't stand a chance against Wyatt's curious grasp. He wanted to hold everything, and I decided that I didn't want to hold him until I was able to have my drain removed.

My five o'clock blood test revealed that my levels were back to normal, and by seven we were leaving the hospital. My nurse had given me a little pink pouch to tuck my surgical drain into at home. The pouch had cream ribbon ties that secured the little bag around my neck. I'm sure it was meant to make me feel pretty, but there is little that can be done to disguise a tube draining fluid out of your neck. It did, however, keep me from worrying about getting the drain caught on something unintended.

We arrived home to a quiet house. Jason's sister Mandie was still watching the kids for us until my drain was removed two days later. Jason took care of getting all the bags into the house, and I climbed into bed and rested in the comfort of the quietness as my family diligently worked to make sure that I didn't have to worry about anything while I recovered.

The next morning, Jason's phone rang early. The stomach bug that knocked me out the weekend before had hit Mandie's family, and she was too sick to keep the kids. I started to get up, but Jason told me to keep resting, that he would take care of everything. Jason went to get all three kids and brought them back to our house. Our babysitter Courtney came to watch them at our house while I continued to sleep and Jason went to work. My bedroom door stayed shut all day. I must have slept well because I don't remember anything until Jason returned that evening.

I ventured out of the bedroom to see the kids and eat dinner. Wyatt started whimpering as Jason was getting dinner together. I picked him up and sat down on the couch. The drain in my neck made me scared to hold him close so I sat him on the edge of my knee and bounced him up and down gently. Something seemed a little off. He wasn't quite himself, and a few minutes later he threw up everywhere. Jason came running in with a towel and took Wyatt from me. We assumed he had the same stomach virus that had sickened the rest of the family.

I retreated to the bedroom and tried to clean myself off the best I could. I wanted a nice hot shower to wash away the day and the thought that a stomach virus was about to run through all my kids, but I had to settle for a quick rinse off. I couldn't get my neck wet until after the drain was removed. So I threw on fresh pajamas, put my hair in a ponytail, tied the little pink bag to hold my drain back around my neck, and sank into bed. I could hear Jason trying to wrestle the kids into their pajamas in the next room. I laughed as I listened to Jason struggle, and I would have gotten up to witness the scene firsthand if I'd had the energy.

The house began to grow quiet as Jason successfully put each kid to bed. Jason came to bed and lay next to me for a little while before he went to check on the kids one last time before going to sleep. I was drifting off to sleep as Jason came back into our room.

"I think something's wrong with Wyatt," he told me. "I put him to bed, but I'd feel a lot better if you'd just come look at him. I think he's breathing funny."

I walked into Wyatt's room and looked into his crib. He was lying in the middle of his farm print sheets surrounded by pictures of little cows, horses, lambs, and pigs. He wasn't sleeping, and as his little blue eyes met mine, his pink lips rose into a smile before he let out a pitiful whimper. His stomach was rising oddly with each breath he took. It looked abnormal, but I wasn't overly concerned. My sister Amanda is a respiratory therapist, and I have called her on many occasions worried about one of the kids. She always asked me if they looked blue. Wyatt didn't look blue, so I assumed he was getting all the oxygen he needed. Still, something didn't seem right.

I picked him up and cradled him in my arms. I told Jason to grab the changing pad off the dresser and bring it to the bedroom. I was a stickler about not having babies sleep in the bed with us. I was a rule follower. Our babies were always put to sleep on their backs in their own cribs, but I decided that the changing pad would keep Wyatt safe in our bed. We laid the changing pad between Jason and me, and I laid Wyatt on it. We both felt more comfortable having Wyatt next to us where we could keep a close eye on him. I was worried we wouldn't hear him if he began to throw up again.

I told Jason that if he wasn't better by morning, we would call the doctor. As we tried to fall asleep, Wyatt began to whimper more. If he had been an older child, I would have said he was faking. It sounded just like a fake cry. Looking back, I know that he didn't have the strength to let out a loud cry, but we were oblivious to what was happening inside his body. I had no idea that a tingling pain was overtaking his body. Jason grabbed his phone and played Wyatt's favorite show "Color Crew." It seemed to calm him, and Jason held the phone above Wyatt until we all drifted to sleep.

The alarm clock sounded and the morning sunlight started to peek through our closed blinds. I thought the morning would bring a happy baby, but Wyatt looked like he was still struggling and uncomfortable. I picked him up and tried to stand him up on my knees as I sat in bed, but his legs were like Jell-O. There was nothing. I immediately remembered how tired I had been when the stomach bug hit me. The walk from the bathroom to the bed had seemed like a marathon, and I assumed poor Wyatt was just feeling the same way.

"Jason," I said. "Look, he's so exhausted that he doesn't have the energy to stand up. I'm going to call the doctor, and I'll make an appointment right after mine."

I grabbed the phone and called Wyatt's pediatrician. I had an appointment to have my surgical drain removed first thing that morning, and I got the first appointment I could after mine. I took Wyatt to his room to get him dressed. His whimpering had stopped, but his stomach was still rising oddly with each breath. I dressed him in new clothes and cuddled him in my arms as I sorted through his sock drawer. As I was closing the drawer, his foot slipped off my arm, and I unknowingly shut it in the drawer.

"I'm so sorry, sweet boy," I said. "Mommy didn't mean to shut your foot in the drawer."

I grabbed his foot and gave it a magical mommy kiss before I put on his socks. Today, I know that he didn't feel any of that. I laid him in his bed and went back to my room to get ready. I threw on some comfortable clothes and made myself look the best I could. I still had the pink bag holding my drain tied around my neck like a medal that no one wants to win. Four days without a shower and little sleep was definitely showing. No amount of makeup could cover it up. I remember looking forward to coming home to a long hot shower after our doctors' appointments.

Courtney arrived back at our house to watch Jay and Austin. I buckled Wyatt into his car seat and grabbed his diaper bag, and we left the house headed for the doctor. We had no idea that our world would look completely different the next time we stepped through our front door.

CHAPTER 3

BROKEN AND BREATHLESS

*I have made you and I will carry you; I will sustain you and I
will rescue you.*

~ Isaiah 46:4b

JASON CARRIED WYATT STILL SAFELY buckled into his infant
carrier through the large glass doors into my doctor's office. Wyatt
looked like he was resting so peacefully that we didn't want to move
him. He wasn't sleeping, but he was so still that we thought surely
he was about to drift off to dreamland soon. I signed myself in and
grabbed a seat next to Jason in the waiting area. We sat together holding hands, talking about what we were going to do over the next few
days. We were blissfully unaware our lives were about to come to a
screeching halt.

After my name was called, we followed the nurse back into
a room where we waited for the doctor. Jason tucked himself and
Wyatt into the corner of the small cold room, making sure that there
was no chance that he would be able to see the drain removed from
my neck. My doctor arrived in the room and told us that my surgery

couldn't have gone better. A biopsy of the tumor confirmed the cancer diagnosis, but the cancer was smaller than expected, which meant I didn't have to have the radioactive iodine treatment. It was a brief moment of relief, and we were excited to have good news.

The doctor finally removed the drain from my neck and covered my incision with a little glue and steri-strips. I had been dreading the actual removal, but with one small pain-free tug, it was over. What a relief! My doctor told me he made the incision in the natural crease of my neck so the scar wouldn't even be noticeable once it healed. He referred me to an endocrinologist and said I would need to come back after the weekend to have blood taken again to confirm that all my hormone levels were normal. He looked over at Wyatt and commented on how quiet he had been during my appointment. We told him that Wyatt wasn't feeling well, and we were going to the pediatrician's office next.

We made my follow-up appointment and quickly headed to Wyatt's appointment. He was still sitting quietly in his infant carrier. I don't remember waiting at his doctor's office, but I clearly remember unbuckling him and lifting him out of his car seat to put him on the exam table. He suddenly felt like a rag doll. His legs and arms just dangled from his little body and his head just seemed a little too heavy for his neck to hold up. My heart sank into the pit of my stomach. Something was incredibly wrong. I undressed him and laid him on the table. I rubbed his little head as I waited for the doctor to come into the room.

Our regular pediatrician was off, so we were seeing a doctor that I had not met. When she walked into the room, I quickly explained what was going on with Wyatt. She leaned over to watch

Wyatt's breathing and listen to him, and as she did, we could see the panic cover her face. She told us she would be back in a second and quickly rushed out of the room. Jason and I just stood there looking at each other.

"You know this can't be good," Jason uttered a few seconds before the door opened and the doctor came in with another doctor.

They both looked at Wyatt and told us that we needed to take Wyatt to the emergency room now. They said it would be quicker if we drove him ourselves instead of waiting for an ambulance, and they were already calling the emergency room to tell them we were on our way. They tried to keep us calm by telling us this was just a precaution, but we were scared and in shock.

I quickly dressed Wyatt and put him back in our car seat while Jason got our van. I literally ran out the front door of the pediatrician's office with the infant carrier in tow. Jason had the van door open and waiting. I snapped the car seat in place and jumped in the front seat, and we raced off to the hospital.

Jason dropped me off at the emergency room door. I hopped out of the van and rushed to get Wyatt out of his car seat. I carried him in my arms as I ran to the first window I saw.

"We were just at the doctor's office, and they told me we needed to come straight here. They said they called ahead and would be ready for us. Where do we need to go?" I quickly spouted off to the man sitting behind the glass.

"Ma'am, just calm down one second," he said. "What's wrong with the baby?"

My voice broke as the words came out of my mouth. "Everything. Everything's wrong with my baby," I said.

I held Wyatt out to him in my hands, and his legs and arms drooped toward the ground. Gravity was too much for them. Jason walked through the doors of the emergency room just as they were taking us back to a triage room. We laid Wyatt on the bed and stepped back as the nurses began their assessment.

Jason and I just watched the scene unfold before our eyes. It seemed so crazy and almost surreal. A sense of disbelief and shock washed over us. We began to tell the nurses what had happened with Wyatt. The ER doctor came in, and we explained how Wyatt had thrown up the night before. We told him he wasn't eating well and seemed to have no energy to move. He said they were going to start an IV and start running tests to find out what was wrong.

Wyatt looked so small lying in the giant bed. He just laid in the middle of it staring at the ceiling in his tiny blue hospital gown while nurses moved all around him. He seemed too calm. There was no fidgeting, no fighting. We watched as the nurse started an IV in his hand. Wyatt never moved. He didn't flinch or pull away. He didn't cry or even wince.

"He's such a tough little guy," I told Jason. "I can't believe he didn't cry when they started his IV." Jason just nodded his head in agreement.

The ringing of my phone startled me. In the chaos of getting Wyatt to the hospital, we had forgotten to call anyone. I saw it was my dad as I answered the call.

"Hey, sweetie," my dad responded. "How are you feeling? Did your appointment go okay? I bet you're ready to take a shower."

"My appointment went good. I'm fine, but something's wrong with Wyatt," I said.

"What do you mean, something's wrong with Wyatt? What's going on?" he asked.

"I don't know, Dad. He threw up last night. He's breathing a little funny, and he just doesn't have any energy. We took him to his doctor, and they sent us to the emergency room."

"You're in the emergency room? With Wyatt?" Dad sounded confused.

"Yes, we're in the emergency room, but you and mom don't need to rush down here. Everything is okay. They said it was just a precaution. I'll call you as soon as we find out what's going on with him," I said.

"Okay. I'm going to call your mom. You know she is going to want to come right now."

"I know that, but I think everything is okay. You guys don't need to leave work right now. This isn't a big deal. I promise," I said.

We ended the call, and I knew my parents would be on their way to the hospital shortly. I told Jason that he needed to call his dad and sisters to let them know what was going on. We didn't want to scare everyone for no reason, but it looked like we would be in the ER for quite a while.

About five minutes later, my phone rang again. This time it was my mom telling me they would be at the hospital in an hour. They lived forty-five minutes away, and I felt like they were probably over-reacting. They had already missed one day of work that week for my surgery. I felt bad that they were leaving again, but I knew there was no keeping my mom away. Grandmas are stubborn like that.

The ER doctor came into our room and explained that they were going to take blood, get a urine sample, and run a few tests to try to find out what was going on with Wyatt. His oxygen stats were good despite his labored breathing, so no one seemed overly concerned about his condition. There was no rush, no panic. They were going to test for something called intussusception. They wanted to make sure that he didn't have an intestinal blockage that made him throw up.

Before taking us for the intussusception test, the nurses got ready to catheterize Wyatt to get a urine sample. Jason immediately started apologizing to Wyatt. We figured it would be painful, and Jason just couldn't watch. The nurse even apologized to Wyatt before she started, but again Wyatt never moved or cried. At this point, I decided that I clearly had the toughest kid on the face of the earth and should nickname him Nails (since he was obviously tough as nails). I mean, what seven-month-old doesn't cry when he is catheterized and has an IV started?

Sometime while we were waiting, I decided to pull out my phone and take a picture of Wyatt. Jason thought I was crazy, but for some reason, I thought it would be neat to have a picture of Wyatt's first trip to the ER.

When we first started dating, Jason's mom would tell me stories about Jason's childhood. Jason was quite the little daredevil as a kid, or extremely accident prone, I'm not sure which. It was probably a little of both. Apparently there was one rather adventurous month where Jason ended up in the ER on four consecutive Saturdays with a different bicycle, big wheel, go-cart, and dirt bike injury. I figured both my boys would be following in their daddy's footsteps, and I wanted to have Wyatt's very first ER trip documented. I had great intentions for making a first year scrapbook.

Besides taking pictures for posterity's sake, I was on my phone searching *intussusception* since I had never heard the word and my son was about to be tested for it. It took me several tries spelling the word for the search engine to even recognize it. I read that intussusception was when the intestines telescope back on itself like a balloon that you've pulled back through the opening and creates an intestinal blockage. I felt like we have pretty much had our share of intestinal blockages, so I was praying hard that Wyatt wasn't suffering from one too.

We carried Wyatt to another room to be x-rayed. He was still limp. I felt like I was carrying around a giant newborn. The test was simple and over quick. Air was blown into Wyatt's rectum while an x-ray was taken. Again, Wyatt never moved or cried. Thankfully, the x-ray looked perfect, and we were sent back to our ER room.

My parents had arrived by this time. My mom immediately took Wyatt from me. She was in full-on Grandma mode, completely terrified that there was something incredibly wrong with Wyatt. I still thought she was over-reacting and tried to reassure her that it was probably nothing, but she didn't believe me.

I got a phone call from my doctor's office shortly after my parents arrived. I had steri-strips on my neck to cover my incisions after my surgery. They're the small fabric-like strips that hold a wound together in place of stitches. They're amazing little things, but unfortunately, I am allergic to the glue that is used with them. My skin breaks out, and I turn into a red, itchy mess. It isn't fun or pretty. The steri-strips can be used without the glue, but the glue gives them a much better hold. When I had my drain removed earlier in the day, my doctor accidentally used the glue, and somehow I didn't notice. His nurse wanted me to come back to his office so the glue could be removed.

I really didn't want to go, but Mom made me. I probably could have talked Jason into letting me stay at the hospital with Wyatt, but not my mom. She was insistent. My dad drove me back over to my doctor's office. He just removed the steri-strips, and gently wiped away the glue from my neck before applying new strips. I felt so silly. It certainly seemed like something I should have been able to do myself.

My dad and I made our way back to the ER and rejoined Jason, my mom, and Wyatt. Nothing new had happened during our absence. We were still waiting for answers. Minutes turned to hours, but there was no change. Two doctors came into our room separately and asked a long list of questions and examined Wyatt.

We were finally told that they believed Wyatt was simply tired and dehydrated. The doctor told us that he could send Wyatt home, but since we seemed so concerned, he would admit him for overnight observations. He expected Wyatt's fluid intake to increase overnight, and he'd be fine to go home in the morning. I'm not sure if we were scared or relieved at this point. Really, we were just tired and hungry. The whole day had flown by, and we hadn't eaten. Jason's dad Walter was at the hospital by this time, and I sent him off to get dinner from our favorite Mexican restaurant. We were going to have a fajita party once Wyatt got moved to his room.

Jason called his sister and made sure she could keep Austin and Jay since we both wanted to stay at the hospital with Wyatt. I think Jason was more concerned about leaving me by myself than Wyatt. Somewhere in the middle of moving into a room, a nurse told us that the doctor had ordered a CT scan. I didn't ask a lot of questions, assuming that the CT was going to be done on Wyatt's stomach.

My mom and I followed a nurse down to an empty waiting room. The nurse told us that someone would be out to get us shortly. I was holding Wyatt in my arms when a technician came out to look at him. He wanted to see how big he was to get the machine ready, and he asked me if I thought Wyatt would stay still while they scanned his head. His head? I instantly felt sick to my stomach.

"Oh my gosh," I said to Mom as I held Wyatt tighter in my arms. "They think someone shook him!"

Tears began to fall from my eyes for the first time that day as a million scenarios began to run through my head. There isn't a person in my world that would ever hurt my kids. Not a single person. My kids are loved and cherished, and my family is amazing.

But what if?

What if the unthinkable had happened? What if there was an accident that I didn't know about? What if he fell over and no one saw him? What if Jay picked him up and accidentally dropped him and was afraid to tell anyone? What if Jason's mom accidentally fell while she was carrying him and didn't remember?

I tried to pull myself together and assure myself that I was crazy. I ran my hand across his head. It was perfect, just like the fuzzy peach it had always been. There were no bruises, no red marks, no scratches. Surely my sweet, perfect baby didn't have a head injury. There was no way, I thought, as I held Wyatt up on the edge of my knee.

But something was wrong.

The baby hunched over my knee was not the same boy he was the morning before. He wasn't squirming and trying to get away. He wasn't trying to stand up and grab my hair. He wasn't even trying to put his hands in his mouth. He was just a limp sack of bones and flesh whose body flopped in whichever direction I moved it. His eyes looked scared and confused, and I was helpless to fix it.

My mom and I carried Wyatt into the CT room and laid him down. The technician asked if we were sure he wouldn't move. I hoped he would, but he remained completely still as they strapped him down for the test. My mom and I went back to the waiting room until the test was over. I wanted to call Jason upstairs in Wyatt's room to tell him what was happening, but I had left my phone up there in Wyatt's bag.

The test was over quickly, and we followed the nurse back up to Wyatt's room on the pediatric floor. Jason, my dad, and Walter had already begun our family fajita party while we were gone. The smells of my favorite foods hit my nose as I opened the door, but fear had replaced hunger, and I no longer cared about the food. Jason knew something was wrong as soon as he saw my face. He rose to meet me as I walked into the room.

"They scanned his head. They think something's wrong with his head," I said.

Jason held me and tried to reassure me that no one would have hurt Wyatt. I knew he was right, but it didn't do anything to relieve the fear that was pumping through my veins. Wyatt laid in the middle of a giant crib while I sat on a couch and pushed around bits of tomatoes, onions, and chicken with a white plastic fork in a room that had become eerily silent while we waited. Everyone was silently pondering their own what-if scenarios.

The silence was broken by the sound of a nurse opening the large wooden door. When she told us that Wyatt's CT scan was normal, I breathed a sigh of relief. Inside, my heart was celebrating, and I thanked God that my baby's precious brain was okay. The relief I felt blanketed the room as we began to laugh and talk again. We didn't have answers, but we didn't care at that point. Wyatt's brain was okay, and we felt certain that he would begin to get better through the night. If there wasn't an injury, certainly he would be back to himself soon.

After we finished eating, my parents and Jason's dad headed home. We tried to settle in for the night. The nurses brought us pillows and blankets to help make us comfortable. We left the house early that morning with only Wyatt's diaper bag in tow. We never imagined that we would end up spending the night at the hospital. I was certain I looked like a hot mess since I still hadn't been able to shower since my surgery. My greasy hair was pulled back in a messy ponytail that made the bandages on my neck unmissable, and any makeup that had been on my face had surely been wiped away with my tears.

I thought about sending Jason home for clothes, but since I still assumed we would be going home the next morning, it didn't make much sense. We could rough it for a night in the hospital. We tried to sleep a little, but it was useless. I kept standing by the side of Wyatt's bed, waiting for him to start moving. I wanted him to roll over. He was a belly sleeper and normally refused to sleep on his back.

He wore me out as an infant when he learned to roll over. The rule follower in me was so worried about SIDS that I would wake up and flip Wyatt over on to his back multiple times a night. All my efforts were in vain because he would roll right back over onto his stomach. I swear I think he even had a little "look what I did" grin on his face every time I found him on his stomach. I finally gave up and let my stubborn little boy sleep on his belly.

I wanted to see that stubborn little baby roll over in that cold metal crib, but he wasn't there. He didn't have the strength to be stubborn. He couldn't roll over or even pick up his pacifier. I watched as his stomach rose with each breath he took. It looked exhausting, and it scared me and Jason. Our worry increased as the night wore on, and we saw no improvement. We finally told the nurse to call the doctor to our room. We really just wanted someone to reassure us that Wyatt was okay. We thought for sure that we would see some improvement in his condition if he had been dehydrated.

His doctor came and put our minds at ease. She let us know that Wyatt was stable, and she encouraged us to get some sleep. Jason and I both finally drifted off in the wee hours of the morning. Jason slept on the small couch next to the window, and I slept in a recliner that I pulled right next to Wyatt's crib. The crunch of plastic hospital pillows woke me with every unconscious change in position.

As Saturday morning arrived, we hoped to see improvement in Wyatt's condition, but there was no change. No better. No worse, and still no answers. Wyatt still wasn't moving, but he was eating and making noises. He could no longer hold his bottle so I soaked up the special snuggle time while I fed him. He smiled at me while he tried to coordinate his suck and swallow, and formula dripped out from the corners of his curved lips and dribbled down the sides of his chin. He looked like a slobbery mess, and I kept expecting him to reach up and grab my hand as I wiped away the formula that rolled from his chin down his neck or at the very least, grab the bottle as I pulled it away from his mouth.

Since our visions of an early morning departure from the hospital were quickly dashed by a motionless Wyatt, I sent Jason home to grab us both a change of clothes. I didn't want to leave Wyatt, but I needed a shower like I needed air to breathe. It had been five days since my surgery, and I couldn't bear the greasy mop on my head a minute longer. I was sure that a hot shower would be the cure for everything that ailed me.

While Jason was gone, I did my best to make sure Wyatt was comfortable and happy. I played his favorite shows on Netflix, and I scoured the pediatric floor and found an infant swing to put in his room. There was no hurry, no rush. There were no procedures or tests. I wasn't panic stricken or crying in a corner, because no one seemed overly concerned. I thought he would just magically feel better soon.

I finally got my shower after Jason returned, and it was glorious. Five days of yuck and stress ran down the drain, and I felt recharged. I didn't even care that I didn't have flip-flops for the hospital shower floor. I was overjoyed to find that Jason had remembered to pack my hair dryer and favorite round brush. I even put on makeup. I was no longer scared that someone might stop by to visit and see me looking like a train wreck.

The day dragged on without much excitement. It was a day filled with waiting. We were just waiting for something to happen, anything, but there was nothing. As the morning turned into afternoon, Jason and I were convinced that Wyatt wasn't merely dehydrated. He had been on IV fluids for more than 24 hours at this point, and he still wasn't moving. We didn't know what was going on, but we knew that answers weren't going to come without testing. We began to get extremely frustrated.

At shift change that evening, a new nurse came into the room to introduce herself and look over Wyatt. She was clearly a veteran nurse and seemed to have a take-charge personality. She leaned over the side of Wyatt's crib and picked up his arm. She let it go, and it quickly fell to the bed with a loud thud.

"This isn't dehydration," she said. "I'm calling the doctor."

Jason and I immediately felt a sense of relief that someone else agreed with us. Letting Wyatt lie in a crib all day wasn't bringing any answers or making him better. There had been no improvement since we walked into the ER on Friday, and we wanted someone looking for a reason. We wanted someone to feel the panic that began to swirl within us.

The nurse came back into Wyatt's room with a pulse oximeter. It's a machine that measures the oxygen saturation in your blood. She was worried about Wyatt's breathing, and she wanted him connected to the machine at all times. She wrapped his monitor around his big toe, and plugged it into the machine. Wyatt's toe now had an ET-like red glow.

A new resident doctor came to Wyatt's bedside shortly after Wyatt was connected to the pulse oximeter. He addressed our fears and agreed that this certainly didn't look like dehydration. He even suggested that it was possible Wyatt had Guillain-Barre Syndrome even though he had never seen a case himself. He didn't give us any answers, but we were happy to finally feel like a doctor was concerned about his condition.

When he left the room, I immediately pulled out my phone to search Guillain-Barre Syndrome. I didn't know what it was, but I knew you are always asked if you've ever had it before you are given a flu shot. I learned that it's basically a syndrome where the body attacks your nerves and paralyzes you. It can cause you to stop breathing and become ventilator dependent. It sounded awful, but it also sounded a lot like what was going on with Wyatt. I read on and was comforted when I saw that most people recover from Guillain-Barre.

Most people recover. Jason and I were good with that. It felt doable and not too scary. We were still unsure what was happening with Wyatt, but we went to sleep that evening hopeful that the next day would bring definite answers.

A different doctor was on call Sunday morning. Our nurse told us that he was a doctor that liked to run a lot of tests. Hallelujah! This is what we had wanted all along. We wanted someone searching for answers. It had been three days since our son had moved, and we wanted answers. We were tired of waiting.

Waiting. Isn't that what everyone in a hospital is doing? Waiting for something. Waiting to go home. Waiting for new life. Waiting for answers. Waiting for healing. Waiting to say good-bye. Waiting is tiresome and hard and often filled with anxiety. We had been waiting for only three days, and we already wanted it to be over. We didn't know then that we were entering a long season of waiting.

The tests were finally starting, and a resident walked in and handed me a clipboard with consent paperwork for a lumbar puncture. They were going to withdraw spinal fluid from Wyatt to test for Guillain-Barre and other abnormalities. She explained the procedure and all the possible side effects. I signed on the line and watched Wyatt be wheeled away to another room for the procedure.

Jason and I stayed in his room. The procedure was quick, and before we had time to worry, he was back with us. The doctor told us that he did great. He never cried, and the spinal fluid was clear. We just had to wait for the spinal fluid to come back from the lab.

So we waited.

A doctor returned a short time later to tell us that everything looked fairly normal with Wyatt's spinal fluid. He did not have Guillain-Barre. We were simultaneously relieved and perplexed. We knew something was wrong, but simply eliminating the possibilities didn't feel like progress.

The day quickly passed as his doctors continued to search for answers. Our nurse told us that it looked like an episode of *House*. The doctors and residents were searching for answers in books and running through every possibility, but they couldn't find an answer. Nothing made sense. Why would a seven-month-old simply stop moving? He was healthy. There was no fever, and he was still smiling.

Finally, a doctor came back to Wyatt's room. Jason asked her if they had figured it out. She told us that they hadn't, but they had spoken with a pediatric neurologist at Children's Hospital in Greenville. Wyatt was going to be transferred to Children's Hospital. An ambulance would be there in an hour to pick him up, but Jason didn't want to wait. He thought it would be quicker to transport Wyatt himself in our car, right then, but his doctor assured us that Wyatt needed to wait for the transport team to arrive.

We quickly realized that we weren't prepared for an extended hospital stay more than forty-five minutes from home. Jason got on the phone and had some friends run by our house to pack a bag for us both. Jason had planned on sleeping at home, so he had nothing with him. It was a frantic hour of phone calls and making sure that Jay and Austin were being taken care of as well.

I remembered that I had a blood test scheduled for the next morning to make sure that all my hormone levels were okay from my

thyroid removal. I knew that I wouldn't leave Wyatt to come back to
have bloodwork taken the next day. I asked Wyatt's doctors to please
help me get it done before I left. They made a few phone calls and
sent me to the lab to have blood drawn. I wandered through the quiet
hallways until I found the lab. I knocked on a door and startled two
workers who weren't expecting to be bothered by a frantic mom at
ten o'clock at night.

I got back to Wyatt's room in time to get him prepared for transport. Even though he was being transported by ambulance, he still
had to be secured in his car seat. (This really made Jason wonder why
he couldn't just drive Wyatt himself.) I lifted Wyatt's still limp body
and buckled him into his car seat. The smile on his face made me
think that he thought he was going home, but it would be more than
a month before he saw home again.

When the EMS transport arrived, I handed Wyatt in his car
seat to them, and they strapped the car seat to the stretcher. I followed them downstairs to the ambulance, talking to Wyatt the
entire way. I don't think he was scared, but it made my mama heart
feel better to tell him that everything was going to be okay. I think
I was trying to convince myself of that more than I was trying to
comfort Wyatt.

I kissed Jason good-bye and climbed into the ambulance with
Wyatt. Jason was going to follow in our car. Wyatt was accidentally
loaded into the ambulance backward and facing the front instead of
the back. Since he was forward facing, I got to see his sweet face the
entire trip to Greenville. He was so calm. The only fear was my own.
I was scared and longing for answers.

The EMT was busy making notes and monitoring Wyatt's condition while we made our way to Greenville. My phone began to chime from numerous text messages from friends and family as word spread that Wyatt was being transferred. I asked everyone to pray for answers. That's all I wanted. I wanted an answer to why Wyatt couldn't move, and in the middle of the night in the back of an ambulance, I begged God to give us an answer.

I told God that all I wanted was an answer, but I lied. That isn't all I wanted. I didn't want His answer. I wanted my answer with an easy fix, a simple solution, and no more waiting.

CHAPTER 4

THE GREATEST OF THESE

And now these three remain: faith, hope and love. But the greatest of these is love.

~ 1 Corinthians 13:13

THE DOORS OF THE AMBULANCE swung open, and I followed Wyatt through a busy ER to an elevator that brought us up to the Children's Hospital. A calmness flooded over me as we walked down the brightly colored halls and past the giant fish tank. I knew this place was where Wyatt needed to be. This place was different. It was made for the tough cases. This place would bring answers.

I followed the EMTs into a corner room where a nurse was waiting. We moved Wyatt from his car seat on the transport stretcher to a new crib and tied on a brightly colored hospital gown behind him. It was close to midnight, but I swear he was still smiling. Surely, he sensed that everyone was there to help him.

Before we were even settled in the room, Jason was there with us. I needed him next to me. I wasn't strong enough to do this on my own. The nurse asked us a few questions and explained there would be a lot of people coming in to assess Wyatt. They wanted to make sure he received the right level of care. Jason and I sat back quietly in the corner of the room as teams of doctors and nurses came to Wyatt's crib side.

We heard things that made us sick to our stomachs as doctors examined every inch of Wyatt's little body. "There's no muscle tone." "There's no response to stimulus." "There's no rectal tone." We heard so much in those first few minutes, and we answered so many questions from doctors and nurses. We went through everything Wyatt could have eaten, everywhere we traveled, and everyone who had been in contact with Wyatt. There were no obvious red flags. His wasn't an easy case.

Jason and I began to feel guilty, like we had missed something, and we were left wondering how we ended up standing in a hospital room trying to recall every detail of our baby's last week. We went through every scenario in our head, but nothing made any sense. Nothing was out of the ordinary. There was nothing different, but somehow everything had changed.

We finally fell asleep in the early morning hours, knowing the next day would be a busy one full of testing and more questions. The nurses told us our doctor would order an MRI in the morning, and again I prayed that God would give us answers.

Morning came quickly. Sunlight poured through the mini-blinds into Wyatt's crib, signaling the dawning of a new day. It was a day full of new hopes and mercies. A day that would change everything in our world. I woke groggy and tired but so hopeful that our new day would be a day of answers.

My mom was in Wyatt's room before we were fully awake. I knew she would be, and I knew she wouldn't leave until we had a diagnosis. She brought Starbucks coffee and a bag of goodies. She's the official bearer of treats in our family, and she's always more than prepared to take care of everyone around her. I was happy she came with breakfast treats.

We snacked on pastries and drank coffee while we waited for an official time for Wyatt's MRI. I decided to unpack our bags since it looked like our hospital stay would last for several days. I hate living out of suitcases. Jason didn't stop me, but I'm pretty sure he thought I was crazy. I put all our clothes in the hospital drawers, and I laughed as I pulled out the clothes our friends had packed Jason. He ended up with a bag full of clothes he hadn't worn in years. I told him this was a clear sign that he needed to make a large donation to Goodwill when we got home.

It was midmorning when we were taken downstairs to wait for Wyatt's MRI. We pushed his crib into a long hallway filled with waiting beds. It was a busy morning, and the hallway was literally lined with hospital beds from head to toe. We dropped the side of Wyatt's crib and rubbed his head while we waited for his turn.

Wyatt hadn't eaten, and for the first time since being admitted to the hospital, he was fussy. It was noisy and a little chaotic. I think the man in the bed behind Wyatt was having seizures, and I was certain that he would fall out of his bed onto the floor at any moment. He saw us trying to hold Wyatt and keep him calm, and in between his shaking episodes, he was telling everyone to let the baby go before him.

Pediatric MRIs are overseen by a doctor from the pediatric intensive unit (PICU) at Children's Hospital. When it was finally time for Wyatt's MRI, Dr. Avant came out to introduce himself and look over Wyatt. As soon as he pulled the blankets back, he saw Wyatt's belly rising with each breath. He was immediately concerned Wyatt's breathing wasn't strong enough for the sedation they typically used. Since he didn't want Wyatt to stop breathing on the table, he called in a team to intubate Wyatt and put him on a ventilator during the MRI.

He explained Wyatt would be put fully asleep during the MRI and would be left on the ventilator and transferred to the PICU after the MRI was over. We were caught off guard. We thought we'd be going down for a quick test, but instead, I was signing paperwork allowing the hospital to put Wyatt to sleep.

My mom had taken Wyatt out of his crib and found a small dark closet in which to sit and hold Wyatt while we waited. Jason stood with her in the closet, and I stayed in the hallway, waiting for the team to return to take Wyatt. To my surprise, a woman popped her head through the doors at the end of the hallway and asked for my mom. It was a friend from her work, and she had come to drop off Starbucks gift cards for us to use while we were in the hospital. I still have trouble believing she ever found us. It was such a sweet gesture and left my mom in tears.

When the team arrived, we kissed Wyatt and handed him off. We were crying, but he wasn't. I think he was too tired to do anything more than survive. We were told to head back to his room to wait. The nurses were going to keep us updated and would let us know once his room in the PICU was ready. We walked back to a room that was eerily empty without Wyatt's crib.

Our friend Jerry, who worked at the hospital, was waiting in the room for us. It was a relief for Jason to see a familiar face. In this age of instant communication, I think we sometimes underestimate the value of physically being there for someone, even when we don't know what to say. There is comfort in being near those who love you, and a text message can never hold you together like a hug from a dear friend.

We didn't talk much while we waited. I don't think we knew what to say. We were all scared, and there were too many "what ifs" to talk about. I opened the drawers and neatly repacked all our clothes into our bag in preparation for our move to the PICU before trying to take a short nap.

After what seemed like hours, a nurse came in and let us know that Wyatt was done. We would be able to see him as soon as he was settled in the PICU.

We followed a nurse back through the large wooden double doors that led to the PICU where the sickest of the sick were cared for. I could feel my heart pounding in my chest, and I was doing my best to keep my eyes straight ahead to avoid looking through the large glass door into other rooms. It was a humbling experience, and I was having a hard time believing that my little baby needed this much care. I was trying to mentally prepare myself for what was to come.

I grabbed Jason's hand as we walked into Wyatt's room. I thought I knew what to expect. I'd seen plenty of movies and even my grandparents on ventilators, but the sight of my son on a vent took my breath away. It is an image that will be forever etched into my memory. He looked so small, lying in a web of tubes and wires. His beautiful face was hidden by a large piece of white medical tape holding the

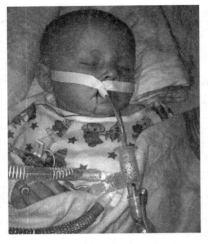

tubes coming out of his mouth in place. Wires were peeking out from the familiar pink and blue striped hospital blankets that covered him when he was born.

He was still completely sedated and looked like a shell of the child he had been just days before. His nurse Anne quickly rushed to our side. She must have seen the terror spread across my face. Anne was a veteran PICU nurse who was truly a gift from God for us. It wasn't by accident that she was assigned to care for Wyatt. I am sure of that. She made it a priority to care for our entire family. She gently explained what all the tubes and wires were doing. She explained all the noises and alarms we were hearing.

Anne was so calm, and her presence made me feel better. She made everything seem less scary. She reminded me that even though Wyatt was sedated and on a ventilator, he was still breathing over the machine. She also told us we didn't need to panic unless we saw her panic. She never panicked and, amazingly enough, neither did we.

The next couple of hours were simply spent waiting and updating family on Wyatt's condition. There wasn't anything we could do for Wyatt. He was asleep, and we couldn't take him out of the crib to hold him. Mom and I just stood staring over the side of his crib. If he started to grow restless and begin to wake, Anne would quickly administer more medication to keep him sleeping while his doctors continued to search for answers.

Jason's dad, my parents' pastor, and an elder from our church had all stopped by to check on us. Jason was entertaining them in the PICU waiting room when Wyatt's neurologist, Dr. Hunnicutt, came into his room to tell us the results from the MRI. I immediately knew the results weren't good, and I cut her off mid-sentence so I could run to get Jason. I literally ran down the hall as fast as my feet would take me and grabbed Jason from the waiting room.

We made our way back down the hall and into the consultation room in the PICU across the hall from Wyatt's room. It was a small, bare room full of broken dreams and shattered lives. There were boxes of tissues and a computer on the counter and a few chairs. Good news happily flows from doctors' mouths at patients' bedsides, but this room was reserved for the hard news and tough decisions. And we found ourselves sitting there in that room of broken dreams and heartbreaking loss.

Nothing has ever been the same since we walked into that room and shut the door behind us.

Dr. Hunnicutt pulled an MRI image up on the computer before us. I didn't know what we were looking at, but I knew it couldn't be good. Dr. Hunnicutt gently and tenderly began to explain that Wyatt had significant inflammation in his spinal cord. She told us it looked angry and went on to tell us Wyatt's body had attacked his spinal cord like a foreign object. She said he had a rare autoimmune response called transverse myelitis and was currently paralyzed.

We heard the words coming out of Dr. Hunnicutt's mouth, but the severity and reality of Wyatt's condition had not sunk in. Yet.

Jason and I sat there speechless as she began to detail the treatment for transverse myelitis. She was going to start Wyatt on a five-day course of strong steroids in hopes that his body would stop attacking his spinal cord. We sat there in shock, unsure what to make of the information presented to us. Then I asked the question that changed everything.

"Is there a chance he won't get better?" I uttered through the tears beginning to fall down my face.

"Yes," she said. "We don't know for sure if he'll ever get better, but I choose to be optimistic until proven otherwise."

Our world stopped.

Dr. Hunnicutt handed me a box of tissues as the drops of tears from my eyes turned to flowing rivers. I listened as she explained that there isn't a true cure for transverse myelitis, but there are treatments. She assured us they would do everything possible for Wyatt. She was so kind and compassionate. She shared with us that she had one other patient with transverse myelitis. It was a young girl who had made a good recovery and was now walking with braces.

Jason lost it. He had sat silently behind me until then, but the thought of his little boy having to walk with braces was too much. No amount of toughness could hold in the fear any longer. Images of Forrest Gump raced into his mind, and it was just too much to hold in. This wasn't a movie or a bad dream. We were living a nightmare. No amount of pinching was going to pull us out of it.

I'm not sure how the conversation ended. I should have been taking notes, but it hurt too much to listen. My brain quit absorbing information and was lost in a spiral of worst case scenarios. My baby was paralyzed, and I couldn't pull myself together long enough to ask the questions I desperately needed to know. I found myself standing next to Wyatt's crib filled with a fear so powerful that it felt like it might consume me at any second.

I just stared at Wyatt in disbelief as I gently rubbed the top of his head. Nothing seemed real. Tubes and wires were coming out of his body, and all I could think was he's only seven months old. Seven months of amazing led to this. How can he never get better? How can there be no cure? How can it be okay for a seven-month-old baby to never move again? How can you be paralyzed in your sleep? How can I take care of him? How can this be God's plan?

I don't know how long we were in this room before Jason finally broke the silence.

"You know we have to tell them," he said. "They're waiting, and they know something is wrong."

He was right. My mom, Jason's dad, my parents' pastor Russ, and an elder from our church were all sitting in the waiting room. I didn't want to tell them, but it wasn't fair to make them wait any longer. I didn't know what to say. Telling someone made it real, and I didn't want it to be real.

Jason walked over and held me, and I sobbed into his shoulder. I wanted to collapse into a heap on the floor, but he held me up and reminded me I wasn't alone. He kissed my forehead and wiped away my tears. He put his hand in the small of my back and guided me back down the hall to the waiting room.

There was no hiding the bad news. It was written all over our faces. I didn't know the words to say. I couldn't even remember what Dr. Hunnicutt said Wyatt had. All I knew was something was wrong with Wyatt's spinal cord. He was paralyzed, and we didn't know if he'd ever get better. Through tears, I shared the news.

I don't remember much of what happened next. I know my parents' pastor Russ prayed. But I can't remember the words. It was all a fog, but I remember telling Mom not to tell Dad until he got to the hospital. He was riding his motorcycle to the hospital, and I didn't want him to have an accident on the way because he was upset. I'm not sure how we told the rest of our family. I don't know if we called our sisters or if our parents just passed on the news.

My next memory is sitting back in Wyatt's room and watching Nurse Anne put the small syringe of steroids into an IV pump. I prayed it would be magic. Anne explained everything she was doing and made sure I didn't have any questions. Wyatt was the sick one, but she treated our entire family as her patient.

I asked her if she could please write down Wyatt's diagnosis. I couldn't remember what Dr. Hunnicutt had said, and I had never heard anything like it before. As Anne handed me back a small piece of paper, she said, "Stay off the computer and don't research this. Just listen to your doctor."

But I had to do more than just listen to the doctor's advice. I had to know what we were up against. I wanted to know how big this giant was. I held the small piece of paper in my hand until she walked away. Once she was out of the room, I unfolded it. Written on the torn piece of white paper were the words *transverse myelitis*. I just stared at them for a while. Jason and I decided we weren't going to tell everyone the exact diagnosis right away. I guess we worried about them researching the diagnosis. I'm not sure how it could be any worse than telling them Wyatt was paralyzed and we don't know if he'll get any better, but for some reason, we didn't want to share it in those first hours.

I pulled out my phone and began to type. T-R-A-N-S-V-E-R-S-E M-Y-E-L-I-T-I-S. My stomach began to churn as I read the search results. This was bad, really bad. Transverse myelitis is a one-in-a-million autoimmune attack, and there is no cure. Only one-third of people with transverse myelitis make a full recovery. One-third make a partial recovery, and one-third make no recovery at all. There was only a 33% chance my beloved little boy would ever get better, and I was devastated.

Dr. Hunnicutt and the PICU team decided it would be best to leave Wyatt on the ventilator overnight in case they needed to do more testing and to give his body time to rest. That meant Wyatt would be sedated until the following morning, and Anne decided that meant I should go home to sleep. I objected strongly. I wanted to be with my baby, but she reminded me I had to take care of myself and Jay and Austin at home. Jay and Austin needed me more than Wyatt did that night, and Anne assured me that I could call and check on him anytime I wanted.

I kissed Wyatt goodnight, and Jason and I headed home to see Jay and Austin. Jason's sisters, Mandie and Robin, had been taking care of them. It was such a blessing that we didn't have to worry about who was taking care of them. Robin was actually visiting from Nashville. She had planned a trip to help me take care of the kids while I was recovering surgery and getting treatment for my thyroid cancer, and I was so thankful she was in town to help.

I called my friend Paula on the car ride home. I told her the diagnosis, and she prayed the sweetest prayer. She reminded me that God was in control and everything would be okay. I wanted to believe, but I'm not sure I did. I spent the rest of the hour-long car ride home

trying to decide how I would tell Jay. Austin was too little to understand, but Jay knew something was wrong with his baby brother.

Jay was only six, but he was the most caring little boy I'd ever met.
His heart was so tender and so full of love. He had seen more than
his share of sickness in his short life, and the thought of telling him
something was wrong with his little brother was more than I could
bear. Jay was made to be a big brother. He cried the first time he saw
Wyatt. He walked into the hospital room and came straight over to
me to catch his first glimpse of this new brother. Jay put his hand on
the newborn's little head, and his bottom lip quivered and tears fell
from his little eyes. He loved him so much, and I knew Wyatt's sickness would break his little heart in two.

Jay met us at the door when Jason and I arrived home. He hugged
me so tightly and asked if I was feeling okay. He had been so worried about my surgery. I told him I was feeling good, but Wyatt was
sick, and I needed to talk to him about it. Jay followed me over to the
small brown leather loveseat and crawled into my lap. Jason sat on
the bottom of the steps facing the loveseat. I didn't even ask Jason
to help break the news. I knew he wouldn't be able to speak through
the tears.

Jay's icy blue eyes looked right into mine as I began to tell him
Wyatt was very sick. He had been studying a skeleton at school so
I explained there was something wrong with Wyatt's spine, and he
couldn't move his arms and legs. I told him Wyatt would have to stay
at the hospital while the doctors worked to help make him better. I
tried to be as honest as possible without going into too much detail
and scaring him too badly.

Then he asked the question I was trying to avoid answering. A question that I didn't know how to answer.

"Mom, is Wyatt ever going to get better? Will he be able to walk one day?"

My voice began to crack as I spoke. "We don't know, sweetie. We just don't know."

He stared at me for a moment as tears began to pool up in his eyes. "Well, we're just going to love him anyway," he said.

I wrapped my arms around him tightly and said, "That's exactly what we're going to do. We're going to love him anyway."

I had promised myself that I wasn't going to cry in front of Jay. I didn't want to scare him, but I couldn't help it. There was no holding it back. With my six-year-old snuggled close, I sobbed until I couldn't catch my breath. I cried for Wyatt and for the innocence and wisdom in Jay's precious answer. He was right. When we don't know what to do next and are crippled by fear, we love. We love until the fear is gone. When we can find no answers and can't make sense of the situations in our life, we love. Love will always be the right answer. When our faith is weak and hope is hard to find, love will carry us through.

Of course, we would love Wyatt anyway. Wyatt was ours. He was our gift, and we would love him no matter what. There was never a question of that, but hearing those words coming out of Jay's mouth reminded me. I didn't have to have all the answers or know what to do next. I simply had to love my little boy.

I had come home to sleep, but sleep was hard to find. Jay had crawled into bed between me and Jason, desperate to be near us. Wyatt was Jay made over. Same blue eyes and round, bald baby head. Same precious smile and gentle spirit. If I mixed their baby pictures up, you wouldn't be able to tell the difference in them. I held Jay as he drifted off to sleep, watching him twist and wiggle as six-year-olds do, and I wondered if Wyatt would ever do the same.

I had called the PICU to check on Wyatt before we laid down for bed, and I stared at the ceiling counting down the seconds until I felt like I could call again. I must have called five or six times. His night nurse was so patient with me and sweetly told me each time I called that Wyatt was doing well and I should get some sleep. I finally dozed off as morning drew near.

My short sleep was broken by a blaring alarm bringing me back to a reality I wished I could sleep through. As I grabbed my phone to call the hospital for another update, I saw I already had a text from my mom. She had already called to check on Wyatt herself and was on her way to the hospital. I knew she would beat me there. I doubt she had slept at all.

Jason and I quickly got ready and headed back to the hospital. We didn't talk much in the car on the way back. We both were trying to mentally prepare ourselves for the day ahead. Wyatt's IV steroid treatments were given every twelve hours. The first dose was given around five in the afternoon. By the time we got to the hospital, he would have already received his second dose. We were praying Wyatt would make a quick, dramatic recovery.

Wyatt was asleep and still on the ventilator when we walked into his room. My mom was standing by his crib rubbing his head. We arrived just before the doctors made their morning rounds. They told us they would be waking Wyatt up and removing the ventilator shortly. They said he should do fine, and we could stay or leave the room when they were ready.

I wanted to see those sweet blue eyes so badly, but I couldn't bring myself to stay in the room when he was extubated. I was too chicken. Jason and my mom stayed with him, but I cowardly waited down the hall in the PICU family room. I was too scared. I was scared to watch him struggle to breathe. I paced the room asking God to please just let him breathe. Moving arms and legs wasn't a concern at all in those moments; I simply wanted the breath of life to flow through my baby. There was such a rush of relief when Jason came to say Wyatt had done fine and was breathing on his own. I could finally breathe again too.

I think my mom may have been more excited than I to have Wyatt off the ventilator, because it meant she was able to hold her grandbaby. When we walked back in the room, she already had him in her arms. Wyatt was on oxygen and still a mess of cords and wires attached to his little body, but he was so content. His breathing was shallow, but he was doing it on his own, and that's all that mattered.

His nurse Anne was working again that day, and she jumped right back into taking care of us all. She got a room for Jason and me at the Ronald McDonald House, and she sent me down to the pharmacy to get hydrocortisone cream for my neck. I had a large rash from the glue that was accidently applied to my neck after the removal of my surgical drain. I was trying to ignore the rash, but it started looking pretty awful. I didn't realize how much I had been scratching it.

I walked to the pharmacy and bought the cream and a large bottle of acetaminophen since I didn't see the pounding headache I'd had for the last several days going away anytime soon. I lingered in the common area of the hospital, watching the faces that passed me, wondering if their worlds were falling apart too. Nothing felt real, and the specifics of the next few days escaped me. Jason and I were scared, the kind of scared that fogs your thinking and clouds your memory. It was the kind of scared that makes it difficult to find the words to pray.

Wyatt looked so frail and tired. Each breath still seemed to take so much effort. I wanted an instant fix, but the more I learned about transverse myelitis, the more I began to realize that recovery is measured in weeks and months, not days and minutes. Transverse myelitis is an inflammation of the myelin coating on the spinal cord. The inflammation prevents signals from the brain from traveling down the spinal cord, just like a traumatic spinal cord injury. The steroid treatments Wyatt was receiving were designed to stop the body from attacking the spinal cord and reduce the inflammation in hopes that mobility would return.

Wyatt's MRI showed inflammation from his C5 to T8 vertebrae in his spine. I didn't understand everything, but I quickly learned a cervical spinal cord injury could leave Wyatt as a quadriplegic. I read all the medical information I could find, but it still made no sense to me. I put my baby to sleep, and he woke up paralyzed. How is that even possible? There is no amount of reasoning that can ever make that okay. Babies aren't supposed to wake up paralyzed. It's inconceivable.

I prayed and begged God for an instant, miraculous healing. He had done it before, and I longed for Him to do it again. Mark chapter 5 tells the story of the woman with the issue of blood. For twelve years, this poor woman was hemorrhaging blood. She was weak, tired, and hopeless. She visited many physicians and suffered at their hands. She spent all she had looking for healing, but her condition only grew worse. She exhausted every worldly option. Men and medicine could not provide healing, but Jesus could.

Jesus was her only hope, and when she heard He was near, she pressed through the crowd gathered around Him and stretched her arm out to touch the hem of His garment. Instantly, the flowing blood dried up and the woman was healed. Jesus made her whole. Jesus asked the surrounding people who touched Him. This woman fell before Jesus, trembling in fear, and confessed what she had done. Jesus called her daughter and told her to go in peace, that her faith had healed her.

This story played through my head as I pleaded with God to heal Wyatt. I laid my hand on Wyatt's rising chest and cried out to God, asking Him to please let Wyatt touch the hem of His garment. I wanted him to move so badly. I told God I wanted Him to heal Wyatt instantly to show the world His glory because that's what you do when someone you love gets really sick. You reason with yourself that it's an opportunity for God to show the world His awesome power. I wanted my Wyatt healed, and I wanted to shout from the mountain tops and tell the world how my amazing God had healed my precious baby, but if I'm completely honest, I was lying. I didn't know it then, but I was lying to myself and God.

I wanted God to heal Wyatt because it was easier. I wanted Wyatt to have a life full of running and jumping and laughing. Life in a wheelchair seemed too hard, and I wanted no part of it. I wanted the picture perfect life I'd always envisioned. Sure, I would have told the world about the amazing healing God provided if it had happened that way, but if God had given me a choice between an easy road and the difficult road that led to His glory, I am embarrassed to say I would have taken the easy road that day.

CHAPTER 5

THE WAITING

*When you pass through the waters, I will be with you; and when
you pass through the rivers, they will not sweep over you. When you
walk through the fire, you will not be burned; the flames will not set
you ablaze.*

~ Isaiah 43:2

THE NEXT FEW DAYS WERE spent waiting by Wyatt's bedside,
longing for the miracle I had begged God to make happen. I watched
every small move and twitch his little body made, eagerly anticipating a drastic change in his condition, but the healing was slow and
incomplete. In just a matter of hours, Wyatt's ability to move voluntarily had been stripped away from him, and I wanted it to be restored just as quickly. I soon began to recognize that Wyatt's road to
recovery would be a marathon, not a sprint.

In the midst of every marathon, there are small victories that pro-
pel the runner to the finish line. Recognizing those small triumphs
is the motivation to keep moving forward, and despite my dislike of
the race Wyatt was in, God opened my eyes to the small wins. Wyatt's

first victory was a strengthening in his ability to breathe. Removing the oxygen tubing from his face gave me a clear view of the ever-present toothless smile still plastered across his baby face. He was still happy even though he was stuck in a body he could no longer control, and his happiness helped bring relief to my weary heart.

Jason and I were also blessed to have a steady stream of visitors those first few days to keep our minds off the reality of waiting. They came with love, prayers, hugs, and an overabundance of food. Bridgette, a friend I hadn't spoken with since high school, showed up with Subway. Others brought bags of goodies. The corner of Wyatt's room was filled with prepackaged snacks and drinks. Trail mix, crackers, candies, chips, and cookies, we had it all. We sent baskets of snacks home to Jason's sisters for Jay and Austin to eat, and we filled the PICU waiting room with a basket of crackers and sweets for other waiting families too scared to leave their child's side to look for food. We still had more snacks than we could eat ourselves, but I gave it a valiant effort as I found sweet relief in anything chocolate. I rationalized that calories consumed in a hospital don't count, but they do. Especially when one day turns into five weeks and ten pounds.

Friends I had grown up with in church came to the hospital as news spread about Wyatt's condition. Casey, Amanda, and Brooke were the girls I learned to pray with in Sunday school, on mission trips, and on the basketball court. We spent many Sunday mornings on our knees together, crying and praying over boyfriends, college choices, and high school drama. Friendships born in Christ are not easily broken by time, space, and the busyness of life, and even though we hadn't been together in years, they showed up when it counted. They showed up, and they prayed life and healing over Wyatt.

Our families were an incredible support for both Jason and me. They held us together and kept life moving when it felt like everything was stopping. We couldn't physically take care of our responsibilities at home and also be with Wyatt. Our families had to fill our roles, and they did without hesitation. My parents were at the hospital nearly every second to make sure we had everything we needed, and my mom took on her role as self-appointed family nurse, questioning every move any medical professional made in an effort to ensure no mistakes were made in Wyatt's care. My sister Amanda was my reassurance at the hospital. She had been a respiratory therapist in the PICU for several years, and she knew everyone caring for Wyatt. Her confidence in them gave me confidence, and Wyatt loved having his Aunt Amanda take care of him.

Jason's family handled our life away from the hospital. They took care of everything so we could focus all our energy on caring for Wyatt. Jason's dad, Walter, managed everything at our office and refused to allow anyone to call us no matter the crisis in those early days. Jason's sister, Robin, came from Nashville to help his other sister, Mandie, who lived locally, take care of Jay, Austin, and Jason's mom. They sent me pictures daily of Jay and Austin on boat rides, drawing with sidewalk chalk, and cuddled together on the couch watching TV, and they helped Jay finish out his first-grade school year. They made sure Jay and Austin were well loved.

By the time Wyatt finished the planned course of steroid treatments, it was apparent there would be no instant healing. Wyatt's breathing had gotten stronger, and he had regained some arm and shoulder movement, but he still did not have any leg movement and wasn't able to use his hands in a fully functional manner. His doctors began to discuss other options and were calling hospitals across the country, looking for anything that might give Wyatt a better chance at a full recovery. They left no stone unturned.

Jason and I are both very aggressive medically, which made medical decisions easy for the two of us to agree on. If there was an option available to Wyatt, we wanted it even if it was a little risky. We wanted to give him every opportunity for what we perceived then as a normal life. We took great comfort in our doctors' search for answers. We were constantly reassured they were doing everything possible, and the PICU staff made sure neither Jason nor I were left with lingering questions regarding treatment or care.

One option available to treat transverse myelitis was plasmapheresis. Plasmapheresis is a blood purification procedure used to treat autoimmune diseases like transverse myelitis. It's a procedure similar to dialysis. Blood is basically removed from the patient's body and run through a machine to separate the plasma from the blood. Then the old plasma is replaced with fresh plasma. The hope for the procedure is that you will remove all the antibodies in the blood that are attacking the patient's body. It sounded scary, but we wanted anything that might provide healing. Children's Hospital had never performed the procedure on someone as young as Wyatt, and after a lot of debate, it was decided that the risk outweighed the benefits since we had seen some improvement in Wyatt's condition.

We were disappointed plasmapheresis wasn't an option for Wyatt. We were still hoping the doctors would find the magic pill that would make everything better. While his doctors were still searching for additional options, Wyatt started physical therapy. We didn't know it then, but physical therapy is essential in recovery from transverse myelitis.

Wyatt's first physical therapist (PT) was a bubbly, young woman named Sue. She was the first in an amazing line of PTs who would care for Wyatt. She had a glowing personality, a contagious laugh, and the best long, curly hair ever. She made physical therapy look like so much fun and less like hard work. She was a ray of sunshine, and she instantly fell in love with Wyatt. She told me she was expecting a little boy, and she was thinking about naming him Wyatt. I'm pretty sure my smiley boy helped cement the name choice for her.

The therapy she began didn't look like much to me, but I quickly realized how much Wyatt had to relearn. Sue sat Wyatt on her lap facing out with her knees together and simply lifted one of her legs slightly higher than the other. She was trying to help Wyatt regain the balance he had lost by making him adjust the position of his head and shoulders. He was hunched over since he no longer had the muscle control to sit up straight, and he didn't have the strength to fully lift his head. It should have been such a simple task, but it was hard work for Wyatt. Sue was the perfect cheerleader, and she showed me from the beginning that the best therapy will always include play for a child.

The days in the PICU were long, exhausting, and filled with busyness. Doctors, therapies, visitors, medicines, and trying to keep Jay and Austin happy at home filled the hours, and there was little time left to think about what may come next. The demands of daily living kept my mind off the demons that were swirling in the back of my head. Life was bearable during the day, but the cover of night revealed the desperation in my heart. My wrestling sessions with God happened in the quiet and darkness of night when sleep wouldn't come and the eyes of the world weren't on me. When the sun fell, my fear and doubts rose.

Waiting for healing, the unknown, is the greatest ache my heart has ever known. It was a feeling of complete helplessness and brokenness. Everything was out of my control. I knew the anguish of waiting from my struggle with infertility, but this was different. At the end of infertility, I knew the results. God was going to provide a child. Through birth or adoption, the end result would be the same. I would be a mom. My ache was born out of my own impatience in God's timing, not a doubt in His provision.

This waiting was different. Staring at Wyatt lying motionless in a cold metal crib, I wept over the uncertainty of it all. Some may call it a lack of faith, but it wasn't. I knew the God who knit together every intimate detail of the universe was capable of healing the child He created, but able and willing are two completely different things. I wrestled with the reality that my season of waiting might just be a refusal to accept that God had said no.

In Isaiah 55:8 the Lord declares, "For my thoughts are not your thoughts, neither are your ways my ways." This verse continued to run through my mind as I begged God to restore my son and make him whole, and I didn't like it. I wanted to run to God and find a refuge from my sorrow. I wanted to use my prayers like a magic wish from a genie in a bottle. I wanted God to lean down and whisper into my ear that a miracle was coming, but He never did. He simply surrounded me with His presence and wrapped me in a blanket of peace that I fought to throw off like a selfish child.

I didn't want peace. I wanted my son to be whole.

I had begged God for a miracle healing once before. When I was twenty-one, freshly out of college and newly engaged, I became a liver donor to an amazing, freckle-faced redhead. He was only nine. I met him at my church daycare where I worked during the summer while I was in school. I know I shouldn't have had a favorite, but he was mine. He got sick out of nowhere and without a reason. He needed a liver, and I wanted to give him mine. I didn't know anything about organ donation at the time. I still don't. I only knew I was the same blood type, and God told me to go, not in an audible earth-quaking voice but in a gentle urging within my spirit. So in the middle of the night, Jason and his dad drove me from Greenville, SC, to Charleston, SC, to see if I could be a match.

It was a whirlwind that could have only been orchestrated by God. I arrived at the Medical University of South Carolina and immediately began testing. By nine o'clock the next morning, I was being prepped for surgery. There was no time to be scared, no time for second thoughts. I was his second liver. His mother had already donated weeks before, but it didn't work. I so badly wanted to give this precious boy new life, but it didn't work either. Two weeks later, my liver failed him as well, and he was given a third liver transplant from an unknown donor.

The third time was not the charm that we prayed for it be, and he never got better. On April 10, 2002, this beloved little boy who had been prayed for by thousands met Jesus face-to-face. His miracle didn't happen this side of heaven. His name was Austin, and I consider it an honor to have my daughter bear his name today. Watching Austin get sick, and then standing next to his family as they said good-bye, was one of the most difficult and heartbreaking things I have ever done. It didn't make any sense. It still doesn't, but I know God was there.

In my naivety, I thought God picked me because Austin needed me, but Austin didn't need me. God certainly didn't need me, but I needed Austin. I could still get lost in a thousand questions about why, but instead I choose to focus on the things I know to be true. In His goodness, God let me be part of Austin to prepare me for Wyatt's fight. I watched a family humbly and gracefully fight with all their might for a little boy they never got to bring home. In moments when I wanted to give up and throw a fit because the cards we were given didn't seem fair, I remembered Austin and his fight.

Wyatt was growing a little stronger every day but remained in the PICU as his doctors prepared for Wyatt to leave the hospital. Wyatt still needed a follow-up MRI, and his doctors decided to give him an intravenous immunoglobulin (IVIG) transfusion in one last hope to boost his immune system. His doctors also began to discuss with me and Jason the options for Wyatt's rehabilitation after leaving the hospital. Wyatt needed to leave the hospital and go to a pediatric in-patient rehabilitation facility for spinal cord injuries.

A rehabilitation center in Atlanta, GA, was suggested to us. A representative from the rehab center came in person to assess Wyatt and answer all of our questions about the center and the rehabilitation process. I am sure the center is an amazing facility, but as I spoke with the representative, my heart felt unsettled. There was nothing specific. I can't give you a single reason why I had reservations about sending Wyatt, but I knew I needed to keep looking for the perfect fit.

I began to look on my own for rehabilitation hospitals. I felt like I was searching for the right school all over again. I fretted over making a school choice for Jay when he started kindergarten, as if picking the wrong school would send him down a path to a life of crime. I was terrified I would make the wrong decision, and that same fear and weight of responsibility felt crushing as I searched the Internet for options. So I sat in the corner of Wyatt's dimly room with my laptop and put the only thing I knew to look for in the search engine: "Pediatric Spinal Cord Injury Rehabilitation."

I didn't even know what I was looking for. Two weeks earlier, I didn't even know that pediatric rehabilitation hospitals existed, and now I was sitting in a hospital with a paralyzed son trying to find one. It seemed unreal.

I felt a sea of calmness wash over me when I saw it in my search results. Shriners Hospital for Children in Philadelphia. This was it, and I knew it. I had been familiar with Shriners Hospital my entire life. My grandfather had been a Shriner in Philadelphia forty years earlier, and growing up in Greenville, SC, I was aware of the amazing orthopedic services provided by the hospital. My niece Morgan was even a patient of Shriners in Lexington, KY, for a hip disorder, but I had no idea Shriners provided care for spinal cord injuries.

The more I read about the spinal cord injury program, the more excited I got. I loved the idea of Wyatt being able to be part of a hospital that would follow him until he was an adult, and to make the situation even better, the spine team from Philadelphia came to Greenville twice a year for a clinic. I knew this was where I wanted Wyatt to be, and I found his case manager at the hospital to tell her I wanted to look into Shriners in Philadelphia as an option for Wyatt.

I don't think she shared in my excitement initially. More than anything, I don't think she wanted to get my hopes up. It's not a given that you get into any rehabilitation center you want. I didn't know that then. You have to meet the center's requirements, and there has to be a bed available for the patient. A full hospital means the patient waits. Wyatt's case manager said she would make some calls to see if it would be possible for Shriners Hospital to accept Wyatt as a patient.

While we waited to nail down the options for rehabilitation, his doctors where preparing for Wyatt's discharge and finishing the final treatments in Wyatt's acute care. Wyatt's second MRI was much less scary. After a quick test to confirm his breathing was strong enough on his own, Wyatt was sent down for an uneventful MRI that revealed the inflammation in his spinal cord was going away. The images looked so much better than his initial MRI.

The news was good, but it still didn't bring any answers. His doctors still couldn't tell us what Wyatt's long term prognosis would be. We were left with the wait and see game, but we knew the drugs Wyatt had been given had worked at stopping the attack on his spinal cord. An additional lumbar puncture revealed more good news. Wyatt's spinal fluid didn't contain any oligoclonal bands. This meant that Wyatt didn't have Neuromyelitis Optica or NMO. NMO is similar to TM but attacks the spinal cord and the optic nerves as well. Repeat attacks were much more likely with NMO. TM usually resulted in only one acute attack in a patient's lifetime. My head was spinning as I tried to read and process all the information I could find on transverse myelitis and spinal cord injuries.

I was waiting for the elevator doors to open, hoping I could escape for a few minutes in a vanilla latte, when the phone rang. I recognized the Pennsylvania area code that flashed on my phone screen. On the phone was Kim Curran, patient care coordinator for Shriners

Hospital. Her familiar Philadelphia accent instantly reminded me of eating soft pretzels and spending vacations with my grandparents in the City of Brotherly Love. She told me there was a spot for Wyatt at Shriners, and they would love to have him. I don't think I could have been any happier in that moment if I had won the lottery.

I didn't know what to expect from rehabilitation, but I felt at peace with our decision to take Wyatt to Shriners. The unsettled feeling lurking in my soul when I searched for a rehab hospital was the gentle whisper of God directing me to the place He planned for Wyatt. It wasn't a mother's intuition or a secret gut feeling or any special wisdom on my part. It was the Spirit of God churning within me when I was looking into options that weren't part of His plan. He was in control even when I was too weak or proud to recognize it.

Wyatt's final days in Children's Hospital were hectic for me as we prepared for Wyatt's transition to Shriners Hospital. I wanted Wyatt to go directly from Children's Hospital to Shriners without going home first. I was scared to be alone with Wyatt. I needed the comfort of a doctor or nurse in case something went wrong, but I couldn't arrange the schedule to get Wyatt immediately to Philadelphia after leaving the hospital. His last IVIG treatment was scheduled for Friday morning, and he would be released later that day.

Shriners wanted to have Wyatt admitted early on Friday or on the following Monday since new patients weren't admitted over the weekend. There was no way for us to make the Friday admittance to Shriners, so we made plans to bring Wyatt home on Friday afternoon and fly out early the following Monday. Wyatt had been in the PICU for two weeks, and he had accumulated massive amounts of belongings in his room. I sent Jason home with a carload of toys, balloons, cards, and clothes.

Jason left the hospital early Friday morning so he could attend Jay's 1ˢᵗ grade awards program at school and get everything at home ready for Wyatt. I stayed at the hospital while Wyatt finished his last IVIG infusion and I signed all his discharge paperwork. I was smiling on the outside, but inside I felt like I was dying. How could I be leaving the hospital with a child who wasn't healed? It didn't make any sense! In an age of miraculous medical advances, I was leaving the hospital with a baby who could barely move, and there was nothing more that could be done for him. It seemed unfathomable.

My sister Amanda was working at the hospital that day, and she sat with Wyatt while I packed the car. Amanda helped get Wyatt strapped into his car seat, and she smiled and happily waved good-bye as we drove off. Wyatt laughed and smiled as he soaked in the sunshine and fresh air for the first time in two weeks. We both could feel the warmth on our faces. Summer had come, but in my heart, winter was just beginning. I drove home to a future I couldn't bear to imagine.

CHAPTER 6

INTO THE VALLEY

In the same way, the Spirit helps us in our weakness. We do not know what we ought to pray for, but the Spirit himself intercedes for us through wordless groans.

~ Romans 8:26

JASON AND I HAD TWO nights at home with all three kids before we were scheduled to leave for Philadelphia. I should have been resting, recharging, and spending quality time with Jay and Austin, but I was a mess. I wasn't a good wife or mother in those days. I was just a pile of broken pieces trying to figure out what I was supposed to do next, which basically meant I ended up doing nothing.

Fear is a thief. It robs us of our purpose and joy, and it completely consumed and paralyzed me. I felt like such a failure as a mom. I had been so confident before Wyatt got sick. He was my third child, and I knew how to take care of a baby—until suddenly I didn't. I was terrified I couldn't fix him if something went wrong. He had an Ambu bag, a resuscitator bag to assist in ventilation, in his bed at the hospital, and I packed it up and brought it home. It stayed within arm's reach at all times just in case he couldn't breathe. He was that frail.

When Wyatt cried, I didn't know how to comfort him. How do you comfort a child who can't feel your touch? I held him as tightly as I could and rubbed his bald little head. He had been given a blanket with red, white, and blue stars while he was in the hospital, and it quickly became his favorite. He had never cared much for blankets before, but now he wanted his blanket tucked under his chin and around his shoulders with the silky tag near his face. He couldn't feel the blanket on his body any other way.

I set alarms on my phone to remind myself to give Wyatt his medicine. The doses of steroids he was given in the hospital were so high that he couldn't just stop taking them without going into withdrawal. He was prescribed prednisone for home, and I was given a detailed step-down schedule to help wean Wyatt off the medicine over the next month and a half. He was also prescribed Neurontin for nerve pain and Colace to help maintain bowel regularity.

Poor Jason went to pick up Wyatt's prescription from the pharmacy the night we got home from the hospital. I had called everything in without a problem. It should have been ready an hour later, but when Jason went to pick the medicine up, they were out of stock in liquid Neurontin and Colace. The pharmacy told Jason it would be a couple days before they had it back in stock. Any thoughts of "What would Jesus do?" quickly escaped him, and it turned into "What would Daddy Bear do?" His heart had never been at a more vulnerable stage in his entire life, and it may have exploded right there in Walgreens. Fear, anger, and frustration collided, and he completely lost his composure.

I thank God that He gave Jason a little self-control. Jason still says it's the closest he's ever come to hitting someone he didn't know. There were tears and a reminder that sometimes customers are coming to pick up prescriptions in the middle of the greatest heartaches of their lives. The pharmacy realized the urgency of the situation and tried to find enough medicine to last Wyatt until we could get to Shriners. Jason ended up at a hospital pharmacy that doesn't serve the public, but he came home with Wyatt's medicine and an aching guilt for losing his cool.

My heart was filled with guilt for leaving Austin and Jay behind again. They had barely seen us in the last two weeks, but there was no way we could bring them with us. I had no idea how long we would be gone or what this hospital stay would be like.

Jay was thrilled to have us all home and wanted to do anything he could to help. He watched Wyatt like a hawk and was so gentle with his little brother. Austin didn't have a gentle bone in her body, but she was only two and was too young to be concerned with Wyatt. She didn't understand anything and simply wanted to be near her mommy. She was already starting to have separation anxiety and was attached to my leg wherever I went.

I could see Jay and Austin's little faces get sad as they watched me packing our big red suitcase that was always reserved for long trips. I couldn't tell them how long we would be gone, and it was all I could do to keep myself from crying. I filled our small suitcase with clothes for Jay and Austin to wear while we were gone. We were blessed to have Mandie watching them while we were in Philadelphia. Jay and Austin loved being with their cousins Addison and Tyler, and it brought me great comfort knowing they would have fun while we were away.

Our flight to Philadelphia left from Charlotte, NC, early on Monday morning. We had to leave our house at 2 am to make it to the airport on time. Mandie came to our house so we wouldn't have to wake the kids when we left. Jay was nestled in our bed between me and Jason, and I tried not to wake him as I grabbed the final bags to take to the car. Jason's dad had come to drive us to the airport. My heart was torn in two as I kissed Jay and Austin good-bye. I longed to be able to be in two places at once.

Wyatt and I slept the entire ride to Charlotte. On top of my concern for Wyatt, I was worried about our flight. I have a completely irrational fear of flying. I realize I'm safer in a plane than in a car. I know that. I still hate it. That's why it's an irrational fear. It doesn't get better the more I fly. I feel like I cheated death on the last flight, and now I'm more likely to fall out of the sky on the next flight. It's insane. I know. I'm convinced it's due to my complete lack of control on a plane, which probably reveals some of the character flaws God was refining during Wyatt's struggle.

I get air sick too. A terrified, air sick woman holding a paralyzed baby probably put me at the top of the list of people you don't want to sit next to on a plane. If I could have justified driving the twelve hours to Philadelphia, I would have. I wanted to drive, but Wyatt couldn't wait that long. Thankfully, Jason was a frequent flier, and he has more compassion than he should with my irrational fears.

As soon as we arrived at the airport, we discovered our flight had been canceled due to "mechanical issues." All passengers were being rebooked on different flights throughout the day.

"Well, awesome," I said out loud while in my head saying something entirely inappropriate.

"Just calm down. This isn't a big deal. I'll get it taken care of," Jason responded.

Jason explained our situation to the ticket counter, and we were the first passengers rebooked onto a new flight. It left thirty minutes later, but arrived in Philadelphia earlier than our original flight since our new flight was now direct. While I was busy pouting about a canceled flight, God was arranging for an easier trip.

Our flight was smooth and uneventful. Jason sweetly explained every noise on the plane to me like I was a young child on my first flight. I just sat quietly, trying to pretend like I wasn't scared. I wanted to drift off to sleep, but I didn't for fear I would accidentally drop Wyatt. He laid cradled in my arms the entire flight. He never cried, just looked around and made sweet baby noises.

Our plane had three seats together next to the window. Jason had the aisle seat, and I sat with Wyatt in the middle. An older, nicely dressed lady was sitting next to me in the window seat. I avoided making eye contact with her for fear that she might want to strike up a conversation. I just couldn't do it. I didn't have it in me. I would have been happy to be invisible. I couldn't explain where we were headed and why we were going without breaking down into a full-on ugly cry.

"That's the best behaved baby I've ever seen. You sure are lucky," she raved to me as Jason was gathering our bags. "I don't think he moved an inch the entire flight."

Jason must have heard my heart break into a thousand pieces right there. Before I even had a chance to open my mouth, he said, "Yes, ma'am. He's a great baby. Thank you so much."

I couldn't speak. She was right. Wyatt hadn't moved an inch. He couldn't. I would have given anything and everything I had to be stuck on a flight holding a baby who was kicking and screaming and fighting to get out of my arms. Instead, as I waited for his stroller to arrive at the gate, I was clutching Wyatt and holding his head like a newborn because he didn't have the strength to do it himself, and I really wanted to stand around stomping my feet because none of it was fair.

My Aunt Debbie and Uncle John graciously volunteered to meet us at the airport and drive us to Shriners so we wouldn't have to take a cab. Both of my parents had grown up in Philadelphia, and my aunts, uncles, and cousins still live there. It was one of the reasons my heart was excited to be able to go to Shriners.

John and Debbie dropped us off at the front door to the Shriners Hospital. As the large glass doors separated, reality set in. Registration for the hospital filled the first floor with a steady stream of families checking in for the day. The back wall was covered with a large, colorful mural depicting Shriners clowns and kids with a range of disabilities smiling happily in a parade. There were children with wheelchairs, walkers, crutches, and missing limbs. We had suddenly entered a world that we had been blind to previously.

I took a deep breath and grabbed a mountain of paperwork from my bag and checked in at registration before finding a seat amid a sea of waiting families. I tried not to make eye contact with anyone and to avoid staring at children in wheelchairs, I fixed my eyes on my own feet that were nervously tapping the floor. There was a young Amish family sitting next to me. The father must have seen the fear painted across my face.

"Is this your first time here with the baby?" he kindly inquired.

"Yes, sir," I answered. "We've never been here before."

"You don't need to worry," he responded. "They are going to take good care of your baby."

My toes stopped tapping the ground. That precious man had no idea why we were at Shriners. Strapped in his infant carrier, Wyatt looked like the healthiest child in the room. He wasn't missing any limbs and didn't have any muscle atrophy. He was a perfect, smiley faced, blue-eyed baby who looked like he was out for a stroller ride, but this gentleman saw fear in another parent's eyes. I'm sure he recognized a fear he had felt before, and instead of remaining silent, he offered kindness. His words were so simple, but I needed to hear them. I needed to hear truth from someone who had been there before.

A nurse from upstairs came down to meet us and take Wyatt to his room. I wasn't familiar with how Shriners Hospitals actually operate on a day-to-day basis. The majority of the patients filling the registration area were arriving for clinic appointments or signing in for therapy or outpatient surgeries. Only a small number of patients are actually treated as inpatients.

We nervously followed our nurse, Amanda, up the elevator to a large room directly across from the nurses' station. The room was typically used as a double occupancy room, but since Wyatt was so young, he didn't have a roommate. I think there was a little fear that a crying infant would keep another patient awake at night, and I was thankful for the privacy.

Our first day was spent getting settled, answering questions, and meeting doctors. Wyatt laid contentedly in his crib, joyfully watching a fanciful rainforest mobile that had been attached to his purple metal crib as a steady stream of people came in to examine him. Nurses, doctors, therapist, social workers, and nutritionists all took their turns talking with me and Jason and getting to know Wyatt. I was struck by the genuine kindness of everyone we met. Despite my fear, I felt comfortable and welcomed.

As always, Wyatt was a little charmer. He had been that way since birth, and he smiled and responded positively to every person who spoke to him. He loved people. He never shied away in fear and seemed to thrive on the attention given to him. At home, he had regularly been the last in line to get one-on-one attention from me. It was simply the fault of being the third child and having a high-maintenance sister and a school-age brother. There was only so much of Mommy to go around, and my never-demanding Wyatt patiently waited for his chance to revel in my undivided attention. He was suddenly the center of attention, and I think he enjoyed having me and Jason at his side 24/7.

I tried to absorb all the information presented to me and adjust to the life we would be living for the foreseeable future. I was struck by the difference in the pace of life between acute care and rehabilitation. The urgency was gone. There was a slower, steady, deliberate pace to Wyatt's care. Part of me hated it. It was especially difficult for Jason and his fix-it-now personality. We were both still struggling to accept that there wasn't an instant way to make everything better, and we felt like someone should still be running around looking for it.

Jason and I received a schedule that explained what each day would look like. Wyatt was scheduled for four hours of therapy daily. He would have one hour each of occupational therapy (OT) and physical therapy (PT) before lunch, and repeat the schedule in the afternoon following a naptime. The evenings and weekends would be reserved for rest and recovery.

My heart took a bit of beating as the picture of Wyatt's rehabilitation came together. We spent the last two weeks in the hospital talking about transverse myelitis and less about paralysis. Suddenly everything in our world became a discussion and an education on paralysis, and it was difficult to take it all in. My only previous knowledge of paralysis were misconceptions from hearing about Christopher Reeve in the media. I learned so much that first day— scary things that gave me glimpses of the road ahead, and a foreign medical language that would soon become my native tongue.

The first big paralysis surprise for me was learning that children with paralysis are much more likely to develop scoliosis and need spinal fusion surgery at some point in their lives. Kids like Wyatt don't have the muscles to hold their spine straight as they grow, which can result in a severe curvature. In order to help prevent scoliosis and provide trunk support, Wyatt was measured for a thoracolumbosacral orthosis (TLSO). It is a brace that helps limit spine movement. We were told Wyatt would need to wear the brace whenever he was awake. Jason picked out a carbon-fiber pattern for the brace.

Jason and I tried to stay positive. The first day was so busy. By evening, we were completely exhausted. Shriners Hospitals prefer to have only one parent at a patient's bedside during the night. The Philadelphia hospital provides double occupancy parent suites in the hospital for parents of inpatients. Jason and I decided it would be best for me to stay next to Wyatt, and Jason would sleep in the parent suite. Since he was the only father staying, he was able to have a room to himself.

I was incredibly drained. It already seemed like days had passed since we boarded the plane that morning, and I wanted nothing more than to find an escape in sleep. In the dark of night, I tried to close my eyes and forget reality. I wanted my old life back. I longed for the simple stress of school and work. I felt like a shell of a person, as if everything within me had been emptied out. I felt nothing in my soul. There was no fear, no joy, no anger. I felt empty and numb to the world around with a numbness that protected my soul from the anguish of our circumstances. I fell asleep wondering why I had turned into the tin man.

Jason's personality is built for the heat of the battle. It's in his blood. He thrives under pressure and makes split-second decisions without hesitation. I think there are parts of him that secretly like a crisis. I, on the other hand, melt into a puddle of mush in the middle of the fire. I was not made for conflict. God was gracious in building the two of us to complement each other's personality. For sure, we are stronger together, and he was the one who awoke ready to battle for Wyatt's first day of real therapy. I might have stayed hidden under the covers if it hadn't been for him.

We were blessed to have been assigned the sweetest therapists. They were truly gems, and they filled us with so much hope. Cheryl Lutz and Danielle Dunn were Wyatt's occupational therapists, and Caroline McClain was his physical therapist. I didn't know the difference between physical and occupational therapy, but I soon learned. OT focuses on fine motor skills and daily living while PT targets the rehabilitation of mobility and quality of life. For those like me—without any medical training and knowledge—OT works on movements of the arms, wrists, and fingers, while PT works on larger muscles and movement like walking. I regretted not studying something in medicine during my college days. It seemed much more useful to me now than my communications degree.

Cheryl and Danielle started working on Wyatt's hand and arm movement. He held his hands in tight little fists and used his hands like claws. He didn't have the ability to straighten his fingers. If Wyatt's hands stayed close-fisted, he risked developing contractures or permanent shortening in his muscles. To help prevent the possibility of contractures, Danielle and Cheryl molded the tiniest little resting hand splints for Wyatt to sleep in. The splints kept Wyatt's fingers together and straight while he slept to help stretch his muscles back out.

I waited for Wyatt to fall asleep, and then I'd quietly try to let down the side of Wyatt's crib to put the little splints on his hands. It was virtually impossible for me to be quiet when dropping the side of his crib. His nurses seemed so stealthy when they did it. I did not. I don't have a gentle touch, no matter how hard I try. I just wasn't born delicate, and after loudly dropping the side of Wyatt's crib, I'd stand as still as possible, praying that the crashing boom didn't wake him before I slipped his hands into the little splints.

He started just wearing the braces at naptime to make sure they didn't cause any markings or skin breakdown before we moved on to his wearing them all night. I was convinced the braces would bother Wyatt since they were essentially restraining the only part of his body he could move, but he never seemed to notice them. He was so tired from working hard in therapy that he slept through the night with no problems.

Wyatt's hands showed an immediate improvement. His clenched fists opened, and his hands became functional. It was such an encouraging sight. It seemed like anything Wyatt worked on in OT was doable the next day. It was as if his hands just needed to be reminded of what they were capable of doing.

PT was a little more difficult. Caroline was absolutely marvelous with Wyatt, but the work was hard. Jason and I wanted to see the same response we had seen in OT, but it didn't work out that way. Caroline started trying to reteach Wyatt to prop himself up on his elbow while he was on his belly. Caroline would put Wyatt in position, and when he was able to hold the position, she showered Wyatt with praise. He ate it up. We all quickly learned that Wyatt loved to be cheered for and he had a strong desire to please.

The therapy was hard work, but thanks to his therapists, Wyatt thought it was play time. A therapist can know all the right techniques to use, but if they can't inspire the "want to" in a child, it doesn't make any difference. A huge part of success in PT and OT is developing a positive relationship with the patient and, in our case, a relationship with the parents. Caroline, Cheryl, and Danielle spent a great deal of time teaching us techniques to incorporate in daily living to encourage Wyatt's continued recovery.

At the end of the first week of Wyatt's stay at Shriners, we had a family meeting. The family meeting involved everyone who was part of Wyatt's care team including all his therapists, nurses, doctors, and social workers. The meetings are designed to give the family a clear picture of the patient's care plan, develop a timeline, and answer any questions. Wyatt's meeting was full of hope and optimism. Jason and I reveled in the excitement each person shared for Wyatt, and together it was decided that Wyatt should have an additional two weeks of therapy to make a total of three for his initial rehab.

While the meeting was encouraging, Jason and I left with a major question: Is he going to get better? That's all we really wanted to know, but every time we dared ask the question, we got the same response: "We just don't know." There was a part of me that almost thought a *no* would have been an easier answer to accept. I could make a plan if I had a solid answer. At least, that's what I thought.

A clear *no* would not have been an easier answer. We were introduced to another patient who had been paralyzed by transverse myelitis several years earlier, and it was agonizingly difficult to talk with him and his family. He was an amazingly strong teenager with a kind spirit. His family was so compassionate and encouraging, but we weren't mentally ready to meet them. He had not made a recovery, and he was the image of our biggest fear. We didn't understand yet that life could still be amazing from a chair.

The weekends were agonizingly slow. The weekdays flew by as I tried to keep up with Wyatt's full daily schedule—breakfast, therapy, rest, therapy, lunch, nap, therapy, therapy, dinner, bath, and finally bed. I quickly fell asleep each night in anticipation of repeating the same schedule over again. Those days didn't leave much time for reflection and self-pity, but the weekends provided ample time for my mind to contemplate the bleakness of my circumstances.

A rooftop playground was located just a few feet from Wyatt's room. It was made like a rubberized running track to allow children with mobility issues to move around easily and safely. Jason and I took Wyatt for walks during our down time. I pushed his stroller around the play area, hoping that the sunshine and fresh air would be good medicine for us all. Then Jason and I would sit on the benches, silently staring off into the distance, both trying to be strong for the other.

I'm not sure what was going on in Jason's head, but I focused on the busy streets below. I was mesmerized by the continuous flow of people beneath me. The noises of the city swirled through my head. The horns, the engines, the sirens, the shutting car doors, the chattering voices, and the thundering roar of the subway below permeated my mind. It was all a reminder that life continued on outside the walls of the hospital. Whether Wyatt was healed or not, life would keep moving, and I had to figure out a way to move with it when all I really wanted to do was sit in a corner and cry.

I had been given *The Paralysis Resource Guide* produced by the Christopher and Dana Reeve Foundation the day we checked into Shriners, but every time I opened it, I could feel my heart begin to beat faster and my chest tighten. I desperately wanted to know how to care for Wyatt. I wanted to be informed, but it was all too much to take in. Pressure sores, bowel programs, catheterizations, home modifications, and so many other things I never wanted to face were staring back at me from those pages. I couldn't handle the reality of what living with a spinal cord injury actually looked like. It was so much more than simply not being able to move or feel. I became consumed with worry for tomorrow, and my mind raced out of control.

"What if he never gets better? What if this paralysis thing is real and permanent?" I asked myself. "How can I carry him when he gets older? How am I going to take care of him, Jay, and Austin? Is he going to need a wheelchair? Where will I send him to school? How can he dance at prom? What about college?"

I couldn't stop worrying. I even justified my worry as prayer thinking if I was telling God about it, then technically it wasn't worrying; it was praying. I must have sounded like a four-year-old begging for candy after she had already been told no. I politely told God all the reasons He needed to heal Wyatt. I'd even list all the things that would be difficult in the days ahead if God didn't heal him—as if He didn't already know.

Worry has always been the vise that squeezed me tightest. I can go from a bright, sunny day to the sky is falling in the blink of an eye. Worry has been my constant companion, especially as a mother who desperately wants to protect her children. I know the Bible calls it sin, but I wanted to hold on to it. It was mine, and I felt like my worry showed God how much I cared about the things and people I fretted over, like He would heap down an extra helping of blessings and protection upon them since I loved them so much. It was a twisted logic, but it justified my desire to maintain control of my comfortable circumstances.

I carried my worry around with me, easily hidden until all my worries became real. I wasn't strong enough to be the mom of a paralyzed child. It was too hard, and looking at the future through the lens of a disability changed everything in my world. Tomorrow became too much bear. The worries of what would come next were suffocating the life out of me, and in the midst of a worried prayer, I felt the Holy Spirit whisper "today."

I grabbed my Bible and searched for the verse that was being branded on my heart. I didn't remember the exact wording, but I knew the passage. I knew the Spirit was telling me to cling to it. It was Matthew 6:34: "Therefore do not worry about tomorrow, for tomorrow will worry about itself. Each day has enough trouble of its own." Oh, how I wish I could pull the trouble out of those verses, but I can't. I can't remove trouble from those verses any more than I can wave my magic worry wand and heal Wyatt.

Crying over Wyatt, I realized my only choice was obedience. God wasn't suggesting or asking me nicely to stop worrying. It was a command, because He knew it was necessary for my survival in the middle of the hard places. Worry can never replace faith, and when it does, we lose the power trusting in a loving God provides. Worry simply shouts to the world that our God isn't big enough. I allowed worry to swallow my faith, and it made me miserable and powerless. As I let that verse sink in and recalibrate my thinking, I discovered the most amazing thing. I could do today, and when tomorrow came, I could handle it too. God gave me my daily portion, and once I began living in the present, I was able to see the joys I was missing.

Wyatt's spirit wasn't dampened by his newfound hospital life, and when I decided to stop worrying about what would happen next, I was able to soak in the joy he shared. His slate had been wiped clean by transverse myelitis. He had to relearn everything and fight for every milestone, and I got to be by his side for it. It was such a gift, but my worry had blinded me to it all. Releasing my worry opened my eyes to the life I was missing. I can't remember all Wyatt's first milestones before he got sick, but I can remember the celebration of every one since.

Wyatt worked hard in physical therapy as he learned to push himself up onto his elbows and lift his chest off the floor. He had been working in the evening as well on a mat in his room. Jason and I would lay him on his belly and place toys just out of his reach on either side of him. It sounds mean, but we quickly learned that motivation is a key to therapy with little ones. We have to give Wyatt a reason to want to roll over, and one night it finally happened.

He was wearing the sweetest blue fleece Mickey Mouse pajamas. They were hand-me-downs from his big brother, and I was admiring just how much Wyatt looked like Jay when I heard him grunting. It was hard work, and I could see it was taking everything he had. He lifted his head as high as he could and extended his right arm as far as it would reach, and with one big push into the mat, his body rolled over onto his back. He laid on his back, smiling from ear-to-ear and completely out of energy. He knew what he had done was a big deal, and he was so proud of himself.

Jason and I celebrated like he had won an Olympic medal. We clapped. We cheered. We cried. We made phone calls. We danced around his room like teenage girls at a slumber party, and then we put him back on the mat and asked him to do it again. I grabbed my phone to document the feat so we could share it with our family at home, and he cooperated and did it again.

I loved being able to call home and share good news with our family, especially Jay and Austin. They needed to hear it as much as we did. I missed them so much, and I couldn't wait to have my kids together again under one roof. I desperately wanted a giant group hug so I could hold my greatest loves close to my heart.

My parents volunteered to drive my van to Philadelphia with Jay and Austin to bring us home at the end of Wyatt's stay. The only kink in the plan was that my sister, Amanda, was expecting her first baby, Izzy, to be born any day. They were all on baby watch at home, and I was anxiously awaiting news that Izzy had made her grand entrance. I hated not being able to be home for Izzy's birth. My parents were definitely not going to miss it, and I was praying extra hard that Izzy would arrive in plenty of time for my parents to make the trip.

Wyatt continued to make slow progress. He worked so hard. Therapy was play to him, and he never seemed to get frustrated when something was difficult. His laid-back personality served him well, and he just seemed to go with the flow. I am convinced it is partially because he didn't know any different. His age was both a blessing and a curse. It hurt my heart to watch him struggle so early in life, but his doctors and therapists reminded me that his age was a benefit to him. He had more plasticity in his body than an adult, and it was possible that his body could learn to compensate for what had been lost if he didn't recover fully.

Wyatt's recovery, although slow to us, seemed to follow the textbook, and it left us hopeful that he just needed more time. His recovery followed the progression of the spinal cord. The spinal cord is broken into four different sections: cervical, thoracic, lumbar, and sacral. Each section is broken down by a number representing each vertebra in the spine. The lower the number, the higher the level of injury. For example, a spinal cord injury between C1-C3 is the highest level of injury and typically leaves a person ventilator dependent with complete paralysis of the body, arms, and legs. The lower the level of injury, the more mobility and function a patient retains. The initial inflammation to Wyatt's spinal cord occurred between C5-T8. As he regained movement and feeling, it appeared that his recovery was simply working its way down his spinal cord. At least, that was our hope.

Jason and I spent a lot of our time learning how to do therapy at home. All of Wyatt's therapists were great teachers. They showed us exactly how to hold, position, and stretch Wyatt. After crawling around on a mat to work with Wyatt for just thirty minutes, I discovered how completely and utterly out of shape I was. The high school runner in me was long gone, and my hospital diet of soft pretzels and cheese steaks wasn't helping matters. I marveled at his therapist's ability to do this all day with patients of varying sizes. I knew therapy at home for Wyatt would equal a workout for me too.

My precious niece, Izzy, was born right on schedule and gave my parents plenty of time to arrive a few days before Wyatt was scheduled to be released from the hospital. I can't begin to explain the excitement that ran through me as I anxiously waited for Jay and Austin to arrive. I stood on the rooftop playground and studied the cars below until I saw my van traveling down Broad Street. I couldn't wait a second longer for them to get to me. The elevator even seemed too slow. I ran down the stairs and met them in the parking garage with the biggest hugs I could give them. I was thrilled to have my family back together within arms' reach.

As excited as Jay and Austin were to see me and Jason, it paled in comparison to the sweet reunion they experienced with Wyatt. There were long hugs, big smiles, loud laughs, and happy hearts, mine especially.

As an escape from the hospital, we decided to take Jay and Austin to a Philadelphia Phillies game. My mom stayed at the hospital with Wyatt, and Jason, my dad, Jay, Austin, and I met my aunt and uncle at the game. Jay and Austin were more excited about their first subway ride than the game. We hadn't been at the game long when I receive a concerned text from my mom.

"A nurse just came in and said she wanted to play with Wyatt. Is that okay? She took him and hasn't come back. Do I need to look for him?" her text read.

I actually laughed out loud. My mom was worried Wyatt had been kidnapped by a rogue nurse. Part of Wyatt's nightly routine was to hang out at the nurse's station. He loved smiling at everyone as they walked by and helping the nurses make their evening rounds. I jokingly called him a therapy baby, because much like a therapy dog, he brought comfort and affection to each person he saw.

We were also able to squeeze in a quick tour of the city with Jay and Austin. We rode on the top of a double decker bus and soaked in the history of a city that was becoming our second home. We passed the Philadelphia Museum of Art and the famous *Rocky* steps. Visitors were running to the top and throwing their arms into the air in victory. Jason looked over at me and without saying a word, I knew what he was thinking. One day. Our dream for Wyatt was to climb those steps.

Back at Shriners, one of the other patients in the hospital was a young boy from Syria. He was an amputee, and he and his mother had been at the hospital long before we arrived. His mother instantly loved Wyatt. When she saw him, she would dash down the hall to be near him. She would dance and speak words I didn't understand.

I could see her face light up behind the black hijab she wore as she reached out to hold Wyatt's hand and touch his face.

I don't know their story or how they ended up at Shriners, but I often wondered if life in the hospital was the safest she had known. One of the nurses told me she had never seen the woman smile the way she did when Wyatt came into a room. While I was packing bags and loading the cart to take our belongings to the van, she appeared in Wyatt's doorway with her translator.

"She wants me to tell you this," her translator began. "She wants you to know that she loves your baby, but she doesn't know why."

I stood there in shock, fighting back tears. I could only muster up a measly little thank you, but I should have said so much more. I failed her that day. It wasn't Wyatt she was in love with. It was the Spirit of God that had been prayed over my precious baby. The Holy Spirit surrounded us, and it was Him she was drawn to, not Wyatt. I still pray for her and her son. I pray that someone else will be braver than I was and will introduce her to the Lord of Lords, and I pray I won't waste another opportunity to share the gospel.

Wyatt's final therapy session was a celebration for our family. His physical therapist Caroline came along with his music therapist, who visited Wyatt a few times each week. Wyatt was usually too tired to participate in music therapy. It usually turned into the therapist singing Wyatt to sleep, but this last day was different. Wyatt had an audience, and he was ready to perform. My mom, dad, Jay, Austin, Jason, and I sat around Wyatt's room watching and marveling at him as he wiggled his little head back and forth and shook a maraca. Jay and Austin joined in the singing, and I did my best to contain my emotions. There was so much to be thankful for and so many reasons to sing. I didn't know what the future held, but my family was back together. That was enough.

CHAPTER 7

HOME AGAIN

The thief does not come except to steal, and to kill, and to de-
stroy. I have come that they may have life, and that they may have it
more abundantly.

~ John 10:10 (NKJV)

HOME SHOULD HAVE BEEN A grand celebration, a return to a refuge and place of comfort, but home was hard. It was like bringing
home a new baby, adjusting to a new schedule, and discovering a level
of tired I never knew existed. Except I didn't have the excited visitors
and covered dish dinners that come with new babies. Home was a
swift slap-in-the-face reminder that life had changed, and there was
no escaping it. Home was a reality I couldn't escape.

Home was full of reminders of the way things used to be. The
jumper in the door hung still. Jay's old walker grew dusty waiting to
guide little feet across floor. The bath seat sat useless in the corner of
the bathroom.

I shoved the jumper in the bottom of the closet. I tossed the walker and bath seat outside on the back deck. I didn't care what happened to them. I just wanted to forget them.

I pulled out all the old infant gear I had previously packed away as Wyatt grew. An infant swing and bouncy seat were once again essential to daily living. Without them, Wyatt could only lie helpless in the middle of the floor and watch life go by. I gave daily lectures to Jay and Austin, reminding them both they had to tell Mommy and Daddy if they accidentally hurt Wyatt, even if he didn't cry. I was terrified they would accidentally step on Wyatt and I'd never know since Wyatt couldn't feel it.

Wyatt's new schedule was busy and often overwhelming. It was supposed to be summer break for the kids, but there was no rest for our weary minds and bodies. We were always moving. We had to be. Wyatt's recovery depended on it. I felt like I was shuttling teenagers around to activities. My Lilly Pulitzer planner had become my constant companion. Its fanciful vacation planning pages mocked me. The calendar was full of therapies and doctor's appointments, and the blank pages in the back were filled with doctors' names, addresses, and phone numbers. Only the weekend squares were blank squares. Wyatt had PT three times a week and OT twice a week. I didn't realize then how unusual it was for a child to have therapy so often.

Wyatt transitioned easily into therapy at home. What a blessing that was! Just by chance, my friend Paula was working at a pediatric therapy clinic called Hands of Hope. I was clueless about where Wyatt needed to be, and so I went to the only place I had heard of in our hometown. I didn't know anything about the clinic, but I knew about the hearts of the people who worked there. They loved Jesus, and He was the hope they longed to give. There were bigger, fancy therapy centers, but none that could have prayed or loved Wyatt and our family more. Wyatt's therapists, Hope, Kim, and Nicole, quickly became like part of the family, and I needed their prayers more than anything else.

Wyatt had another IVIG treatment a couple weeks after we returned home. It was an additional effort on his doctor's part to boost his recovery, and we were hoping to see a definitive response from the procedure. The IVIG was done at an outpatient pediatric infusion center. It sounds fancy, but it was just a room full of chairs in a doctor's office. The sight of the room left me anxious. There were no cribs, only large, uncomfortable recliners, and I would have to hold Wyatt on my lap for 4-6 hours. I'm glad Jason had come with us, because I felt completely unprepared to keep Wyatt entertained.

The nurses had trouble getting Wyatt's IV started. I preferred to have the IV in his foot since he couldn't move or feel it. It seemed to make the most sense, but it just wouldn't work. After several failed attempts on his arms as well, a nurse told me we may need to reschedule because she couldn't stick his arms again. I wasn't taking Wyatt home without the treatment he had come to get, so I suggested his head. He was bald and you could perfectly see all the veins running along the side of his head. An IV was never placed in his head during his PICU stay, but it had been suggested as an option. The nurse agreed, and with one quick stick, the IV was in.

The IV looked awful coming out of the side of his head, but it was the perfect solution for Wyatt. It was out of sight and out of mind. He completely forgot it was there, and it kept him free to move his arms without any restraint. My mom came to help us entertain Wyatt. I'm so glad she didn't listen to me when I told her the night before she didn't need to come. Jason and I definitely needed the help.

We took turns holding Wyatt and trying to get him to sleep. After a couple hours, I left Wyatt in my mom's arms and went to grab a bite to eat in the lobby. Before I could get back, Jason met me in the hall outside the doctor's office. He wanted to prepare me for the horror-like scene that ensued after I left. My mom had been bouncing Wyatt on her lap and inadvertently knocked the IV out, and a lot of blood had streamed from his little head and covered him and my mom. All the excitement was over by the time I returned, and the nurses were putting a new IV in the other side of his head to finish his treatment. My poor mom was so upset and felt incredibly guilty. Jason still loves to tease her about it.

The adjustment to our new life was much easier for Wyatt, Jay, and Austin than it was for me. They were so flexible and just went with the flow. I was smiling on the outside, but on the inside, part of me was dying. Loneliness consumed me, and I felt isolated in a world no one else could understand. The text messages and phone calls stopped once Wyatt came home from the hospital, but I needed them more than ever. I'm not sure why it happened that way. Maybe it was because Wyatt didn't look different and people couldn't see what he had lost. Maybe I did a poor job conveying the seriousness of his condition, or maybe I looked like I had it all together. Whatever the reason, Jason and I felt like we had been forgotten. We were grounded in our faith, but we still struggled to hold it all together.

Each day, I prayed for enough strength to make it through without falling apart. I didn't know how to control the emotions pouring out of me. I had never been overly emotional before. I guess I thought

I was tough. I remember joking with Jason during our wedding because he couldn't stop crying and I didn't shed a tear. Now I had lost my strong exterior shell. I was reduced to a soft, weepy mess and often found myself hiding behind a closed bathroom door to keep the kids from witnessing me in such a devastated state.

I needed a way to process all the emotions I was experiencing, and I longed for a way to connect with other people experiencing similar situations. I found community through social media. Facebook was suddenly more than a brag book and highlight reel. It was a resource that provided real-life information. I found groups for parents of children with TM and groups for sufferers of TM, and they shared my hurts. They knew my pain, and the island I was stuck on didn't seem so isolating. I found real advice from others living through the same storms. I found a place to ask all the crazy questions running through my head.

On a whim, I created Wyatt's Fight Against TM on Facebook. In hindsight, I should have chosen a shorter name, but I didn't know any better. I wanted a place to share and document Wyatt's recovery, and I wanted a way to easily connect with other families struggling through TM or spinal cord injuries. I didn't know his Facebook page would soon become my therapy and a place to pour out my heart.

Jason was not fond of the Facebook page in the beginning. He is very particular in the information he chooses to share with others, but I typically don't have an unspoken thought. We couldn't be more different like that. It drives him crazy. If you met us in person, you'd believe it was the other way around. Jason is a true extrovert, always approachable and never without a warm smile. He's always friendly and ready to strike up a conversation, while I struggle mightily to make one-on-one conversation, but Jason guards what he says. He never wants to appear to be complaining about life.

I think Jason is terrified of looking ungrateful. He hates asking for prayer for the little things. I am convinced that part of him comes from growing up in a Baptist church where members regularly asked for "traveling mercies" for cruises and fun vacations. Prayer time could sound like a gossip fest, and Jason never wanted any part of it. He was worried Wyatt's Facebook page would turn into a giant pity party, but he went along with my idea despite his concerns.

As I kept Wyatt's Facebook page updated, I saw my own newsfeed filled with summertime fun. I scrolled through picture after picture of families frolicking in the ocean and building towering sandcastles, and I was jealous. I became determined to do something I considered normal, and in a moment of temporary insanity, I decided that we needed to take the kids to the beach before school started back.

Jason hates all things beach. The heat. The sand. Carrying nine million things to the ocean daily. A day at the beach looks a whole lot like work to Jason. He'd been able to avoid a beach vacation for our entire marriage, but he didn't have the heart to tell me no any longer. I played the guilt card. Jay's birthday was coming up, and I felt guilty for not throwing him a fancy Pinterest party. I told Jason we needed to take Jay to the beach to make up for all he'd been through during the summer. Jason caved in. We loaded everyone into the minivan and headed to Fripp Island.

We were ill-equipped for the beach. We didn't have a wagon, an expensive cooler, a big umbrella, or fancy chairs. We hit the beach with only towels, a boogie board, and a bucket with a shovel, and it was perfect. Jay and Austin came to life as soon as their feet hit the sand and their lungs filled with salty air. They soaked up being the center of our attention. So much of their summer had been spent waiting in doctor's offices. It was refreshing to watch them splash and play carefree in the ocean. Jay loved being in the ocean with Jason and riding the boogie board. Austin was obsessed with digging in the sand. She even made sure Wyatt had a shovel to hold as he watched.

I wasn't ready to head home after such a great weekend. The beach let me forget about the all-consuming schedule I had been keeping, so we extended our stay even though Jason had to leave to work during the day. A crazy set of circumstances left me taking care of Jason's mom at the beach as well. I'm not sure what made me think taking a paralyzed baby, an Alzheimer's patient who had a colostomy, and two other children to the ocean was a good idea, but I did it.

I carried Wyatt in a baby carrier on my chest and threw beach bags over my shoulder. I gave Jason's mom all the beach toys to hold. Jay carried a Bumbo seat for Wyatt and held Austin's hand. Together, we hiked to the beach. The five-minute walk took us at least twenty minutes. It was a miracle we made it without anyone falling or crying. I could have hugged the boy at the umbrella stand. I rented an umbrella and chairs for the day, and when I finally had everyone settled, I sat down in the shade and prayed no one would ask to go to the bathroom. Thankfully, God had mercy on us, and we had a problem-free day. I couldn't have planned it better. We were even able to get a cake and celebrate Jay's seventh birthday that night. It really was such a blessing to have time away from doctors and therapists and recharge before the kids returned to school.

I wanted life to be as normal as possible for Wyatt, so we enrolled him in the same preschool he had attended before he got sick. The staff loved Wyatt and was more than willing to accommodate him in any way possible. I didn't want to isolate him at home, and I thought being around other children his age would encourage him to move and help his recovery. Since his birthday is in September, he was the oldest child in the class, and his paralysis wasn't an obvious difference since his classmates weren't walking yet.

Wyatt's therapist started visiting him at school, and I tried to go back to work as much as possible. We were developing a routine. It was a crazy routine, but at least there was a little consistency to our days. Frozen pizza and chicken nuggets became our staple for dinner. We were in a survival season, and we threw out every expectation about what life should look like. Encouraging Wyatt to continue therapy as part of our everyday living was our family priority. Even Jay and Austin were excited to watch Wyatt relearn the smallest task. We all knew Wyatt's recovery would be a slow process, but we continued to be encouraged that a recovery was on its way. I even joked that ESPN always needed a great backstory, and this healing would be Wyatt's.

A few weeks after school started, Wyatt had a follow-up MRI. Jason and I weren't concerned about it at all. I figured it was just routine, and I didn't expect to get any new information. His previous MRI had shown the inflammation in his spinal cord had gone down, and I knew it hadn't gotten any worse. I was only worried about Wyatt waking up cranky from the anesthesia after the MRI was over. I didn't give the results a second thought.

We arrived at Children's Hospital and went straight back to prepare for the MRI. We saw a lot of familiar faces who were shocked at how much better Wyatt looked. He was a different child than the one who just months before was struggling to breathe during his first MRI.

A nurse we had never met came in to get Wyatt ready for the MRI. As she leaned over Wyatt, listening to his heart and lungs, she offhandedly told him he better not kick her in the face.

"Wyatt, if you kick her in the face, I will buy you a car on the way home," Jason chimed in without missing a beat.

The nurse looked up at Jason completely shocked and dumbfounded.

"Excuse me?" she said, confused.

"He's paralyzed. We'd love for him to be able to kick you," Jason informed her.

She began to apologize profusely, but Jason and I just laughed. We had learned not to take things too seriously. Wyatt went back for an uneventful MRI, and I swear he woke up smiling. I'd like to say he was smiling at me, but I am sure the smile was for the bottle I was holding. We all left the hospital surprised at how easy the process had been.

Wyatt was in the middle of therapy the following day when I received a call from Wyatt's doctor's office. I was surprised when I heard Dr. Hunnicutt's voice. I was impressed she called me herself, but the words that followed cut my heart in two and tested everything I believed.

"I've looked over the results of Wyatt's MRI," she began. "I'm so sorry to tell you this, but Wyatt isn't going to be someone who makes a full recovery. There is narrowing in his spinal cord. It looks similar to the waistline of a Barbie doll."

Dr. Hunnicutt's words were compassionate, but there was no way to soften the blow. The TM attack had eaten away a portion of his spinal cord, and there was nothing medicine could do to repair it. I didn't know how to respond. I had no idea this was even a possibility. All I could do was cry.

I tried to pull myself together long enough to call Jason. Through tears, I managed to tell Jason the test results. The shock hit him too, but he did his best to console me.

"Abby, you have to calm down," he told me. "It's going to be okay. We can do this. No one knows what may happen down the road. Wyatt is going to have a great life. I know it. We just have to keep working hard for him and for Jay and for Austin. I promise. It's all going to be okay."

He was trying to convince himself as much as he was trying to convince me. *Okay* was such a relative term. Everyone liked to throw it around like it was a bandage for my bleeding heart, but okay didn't fix anything. I wanted good, amazing, or extraordinary. I didn't want to settle for a life of just okay for myself or Wyatt.

I walked back into the room where Wyatt was having therapy, and I shared the devastating news with Wyatt's therapist Hope and my friend Paula. They stopped everything and instantly began praying over Wyatt's life. They prayed for strength and wisdom, and they reminded me that my hope is not in medicine. My hope is in Jesus Christ.

I wrestled with God that night. I had accepted the path we were on as long as it meant healing for Wyatt in the end. I didn't care how long the journey would take. The fight was worth the effort if Wyatt's body was restored. I wasn't ready to embrace suffering for suffering's sake. I wanted it to be worth something.

I cried out to God, begging Him to a make a way. I pleaded for the God of the Universe, the Creator of the Stars, the One who perfectly formed Wyatt in my womb and knew the number of hairs on his head, to send the healing Wyatt was waiting for. I was waiting for a profound answer to fall from the heavens when I felt a nudge from the Holy Spirit telling me to quit waiting. Wyatt wasn't waiting. I was the one waiting, and it wasn't what God had ever intended for me.

I was waiting for life to be perfect, to look like the picture I had planned. I wasn't just waiting for healing. I was waiting to live. I had put everything on hold, which had been a constant pattern in my life. I had always been waiting for something. Waiting to get married. Waiting to have children. Waiting for our company to grow. Waiting for a bigger house. I was always waiting for the next thing I thought would make my life better or easier.

God's Word repeatedly tells us to wait on Him, but I wasn't waiting on Him. I was waiting on what He could do for me. I was waiting for God to change my circumstances and make my life more comfortable. I spent so much time waiting on what I wanted that I was missing the goodness before me. At some point, the crying has to end so living can begin. Time was not waiting for me, and despite his struggles, Wyatt loved the life he was living, and I knew I had to love it too.

I get only one chance to be Wyatt's mom, and I don't want him growing up believing I am more concerned about the wholeness of his body than the holiness of his heart. I had been living a life dictated by my circumstances instead of the God who controls them. I decided while lying in bed that night that tomorrow was a new day, and I was going to bask in the mercies the Lord provided. I would celebrate the life God had given me and Wyatt, and I would not let my joy be diminished by the muck I was wading through. God was bigger than it all.

The next morning, the sun rose just as it had every day since Wyatt became paralyzed, but it seemed brighter. I got the kids up and started getting them ready for school. We laughed and played and even made it to school on time, which was a huge deal for my habitually late family. I didn't know how I was going to stay positive, but I was determined to quit living a negative life. So I did the only thing I knew to do: the next thing. Sometimes the next thing was simply getting the kids ready for school, and that's what I did. I did whatever came next, and I tried to do it with a smile.

Learning Wyatt's paralysis was likely permanent didn't change his treatment plan. First Corinthians 6:10 says that our bodies are a temple of the Holy Spirit. If the temple falls or is damaged, you rebuild it. You don't throw your hands up in the air and give up. Jason and I weren't going to give up on Wyatt walking one day, no matter what his MRI showed. Wyatt's therapy wasn't just about walking. It was about making and keeping him healthy. Therapy is like exercise, and it was essential for Wyatt to work hard to maintain the muscles he had. We weren't about to stop working and let his muscles waste away or atrophy.

I continued to read and study all I could find on paralysis and spinal cord injuries. Jason and I truly believe there will be a cure for paralysis in Wyatt's lifetime. We don't know when or how, but we believe it will come. We take it as our job to make sure he is healthy enough to take advantage of it when it becomes available. If a cure is discovered when Wyatt is twenty-five, but we have let his muscles waste away and atrophy, it will do no good for him. I don't want Wyatt to ever look back as an adult and think, "If only Mom and Dad had done this differently, I would be walking today." I wanted to be educated on Wyatt's condition and all the opportunities and clinical trials available to him.

I asked other parents of TM kids for advice. I wanted to know what they would do differently from the beginning and what treatments or therapies they would recommend. I knew my best resource would be parents fighting this battle. Across the board, I was encouraged to research neuromuscular electrical stimulation (NMES) and the Kennedy Krieger Institute (KKI). NMES is a treatment that uses a device to transmit electrical currents to select muscle groups through electrodes placed on the skin. The current creates a shock that causes the selected muscles to contract, making it a valuable tool for spinal cord injury patients to exercise muscles they no longer have control over.

KKI is a pediatric rehabilitation hospital in Baltimore, MD, and home to the International Center for Spinal Cord Injury. I researched it online. It looked like an amazing facility with state-of-the-art equipment and world class doctors, but I didn't understand how rehabilitation stays worked. Wyatt hadn't been home from Shriners Hospital long, and I didn't think another inpatient hospital stay would be available to him. I just filed the information about KKI in the back of my mind and started to pursue NMES for Wyatt.

I mentioned it to Wyatt's therapist. His OT, Nicole, just happened to have a NMES unit he could use! I had also begun to notice Wyatt was developing a worsening foot drop. Foot drop is a general term that refers to the inability to lift the front part of the foot. Someone who walks and experiences foot drop might drag their toes and be susceptible to falls. When I looked at Wyatt's feet, his toes always appeared to be pointing down, and his foot was never at a 90-degree angle. Obviously, I wasn't worried about him tripping or dragging his toes since he wasn't walking, but foot drop is significant for those living with paralysis because it can cause the muscles to permanently tighten, resulting in a foot that won't bend into a normal position. Braces called ankle-foot orthosis (AFO) are used to hold the foot in the correct position and prevent foot drop.

Wyatt was referred to Shriners Hospital in Greenville, SC, to have his AFOs made. He had to be seen and accessed by a doctor in Greenville, and during his initial clinic visit, he was also seen by a PT. I briefly discussed Wyatt's history with the PT and mentioned I was interested in learning more about NMES. He had been using it a little, but I wasn't sure how often he should use it or what the strength of the current should be. The PT said she wasn't familiar with NMES herself but would look into it for me.

We were slowly building quite a stock of medical equipment at home. I discovered children outgrow a lot of equipment before they can wear it out, and a lot of good quality used equipment is available through online sale websites and exchanges. I was able to find a stander free of charge from the SC Assistive Technology Exchange Program. One additional benefit of finding used equipment is the ability to have it immediately. Ordering and processing through insurances can take months, and I was able to have the stander in our house a few days after I found it. A stander is a rigid frame that holds a patient in place in a secure, upright position. The stander is necessary for weight-bearing, which is needed for bone and muscle growth.

I received a phone call from the PT who saw Wyatt in Greenville a few days after his appointment. She had been talking to other PTs regarding the NMES I had asked about, and one of the other PTs had previously worked at KKI and recommended it to her. She asked if it would be okay for her to call KKI on our behalf and make a referral. I said yes without hesitation.

Things fell into place, and Wyatt was approved for an inpatient rehabilitation stay at KKI in September of 2013, four months after becoming paralyzed. It sounds completely backwards to say Jason and I were excited about Wyatt's hospital stay, but we were. We were so excited about the possibilities it could bring for him, and the more I read, the more eager I became. We were told his stay would last between four to six weeks, and the difficult part for us was determining the logistics of being separated for more than month.

CHAPTER 8

NEW BEGINNINGS

Forget the former things; do not dwell on the past. See, I am
doing a new thing! Now it springs up; do you not perceive it? I am
making a way in the wilderness and streams in the wasteland.

~ Isaiah 43:18–19

JASON AND I DECIDED IT made the most sense for me to stay at KKI with Wyatt, and he would stay home to care for Jay and Austin. I was more comfortable with all Wyatt's medical needs. On paper, it didn't sound like a big deal. In reality, it was a huge deal. Separation is hard, especially with little ones. Jay was seven, and Austin was only two and not yet potty-trained. Jason was an amazing father, but he had never been left alone with our kids for more than a few hours at a time. He could spend all day alone with Jay, but the little ones still scared him. Diapers and uncontrollable crying just weren't his thing. He pretended like the thought of watching Jay and Austin alone didn't bother him, but I know deep down he was terrified.

The days leading up to Wyatt's hospitalization were full of preparation. Grocery shopping, laundry, cleaning, and packing. I had a huge to-do list. I wanted to make sure Jason had everything he needed to make life as easy as possible for him, Jay, and Austin while I stayed in Baltimore with Wyatt. It wasn't a have-to list. It was a want-to list. Jason certainly would have taken care of everything himself, but I wanted him to know how much I appreciated him and everything he did for our family. As difficult as Wyatt's situation was for me, I knew the stress on Jason was even greater since he was also responsible for keeping our family business rolling.

Again our extended families rose to the occasion to fill in the gaps and help with childcare for Jay and Austin. I never once had to worry about who would care for them in our absence. We had a "Have Baby, Will Travel" attitude when it came to any medical treatment for Wyatt, and that would not have been possible without our families' continued support. Our parents and sisters were more than willing to do anything necessary to help. We even made plans for my parents to go to KKI so I could come home and spend a long weekend with Jay and Austin. We thought an entire month was just too long for me to be away from them. They needed their mama, and it was obvious Austin already had some separation anxiety.

Leaving for KKI was a completely different feeling than leaving for Shriners just four months earlier. Jason and I weren't filled with fear. We were filled with the excitement of possibilities, wonderful possibilities. We fully believed God had orchestrated the trip we were about to take, and we were expecting something amazing to happen. We wanted KKI to change Wyatt's world for the better, but we had no idea about the world of possibilities that would be opened.

Jason and I had a smooth nine-hour trip from Greenwood to Baltimore with Wyatt. Jason drove the entire way since the speed of my driving probably would have turned the trip into an eleven-hour adventure. Wyatt was perfect. There were no major meltdowns or hours of uncontrollable crying. He seemed so much older than his mere eleven months. We were able to check into the Ronald McDonald House (RMH) the night before Wyatt was to be admitted, and Jason was able to stay at the RMH until he returned home five days later.

I'd be lying if I said I didn't have a few fears and reservations about Wyatt's stay. I certainly did, but I kept them to myself because they sounded so selfish. I was worried about my own comfort. The thought of sleeping on a pull-out bed, using a shared bathroom down the hall, and sharing a double occupancy room didn't sound like fun to me. It sounded a lot like the worst parts of college, but I knew voicing those concerns made me sound like a spoiled brat. Wyatt was about to get an opportunity that many others never have access to, and I was determined to see the good in it even if it was uncomfortable for me. While I was excited for Wyatt, I tried to bury the looming dread swirling through my mind.

Jason and I checked Wyatt into KKI on a Monday morning. The process couldn't have gone any smoother. We were even impressed by the kindness of the parking attendant, which gave us a wonderful first impression. We pushed Wyatt around the first floor lobby while we waited to be escorted upstairs to Wyatt's room. Jason and I felt at ease and had an overwhelming sense of relief that we had made it. The opportunity we had been praying for was actually happening, and we were eager for it to begin.

We lucked out again and were assigned the sweetest nurse named Erika. She was thrilled to have Wyatt and reaffirmed our belief that he was indeed the cutest baby on the face of the earth.

We already knew from previous experience that our first day would be full of meetings and assessments for Wyatt. We went over his medical history and medications. We met his PT Sarah Murdoch and OT Kaitlin MacDonald and spent the day getting settled in. I unpacked and tried to make his half of the room feel comfortable and homey since it would be his home for the foreseeable future.

Wyatt's room was directly across the hall from the parents' lounge where the showers, bathroom, and—most importantly—coffee were located. Coffee had become my addiction, and having unlimited access to it a few feet from my room was a welcome surprise. The parents' lounge was actually off limits to children and medical staff. It wasn't fancy, but it was a place for parents to retreat, relax, and vent frustrations if needed, free from the ears of doctors and nurses.

I was immediately impressed with how KKI went above and beyond expectations to make sure parents and caregivers were comfortable. I had to sleep on a pull-out chair, but I was given a foam egg crate mattress pad to make me more comfortable. It made a huge difference and kept me from being a tired, cranky mama. The nurses were always checking on me just as much as they were Wyatt. There were also weekly catered parents' dinner on Tuesday nights. I was often reminded that rehabilitation involved the entire family, and I had to take care of myself as well. I felt silly for worrying about my own comfort.

We were introduced to the therapy center playroom at KKI on the first day. I use the term *playroom* loosely because it provided much more than play. Play is more than a way to pass time. Play is therapy for children, and it's the way they learn and discover their world. Toys were always the motivation for Wyatt to move. KKI had a staff of therapeutic recreation specialists, and each day in between his normal therapies, Wyatt was scheduled time for therapeutic where the staff would reinforce the goals outlined by his PT and OT. The playroom was also open in the evening, and I was able to bring Wyatt down for a time of supervised play while I ate dinner or caught up on office work. I didn't realize how much I needed the alone time for my own mental well-being. It was a gift to me, and it let Wyatt interact with other children facing similar struggles.

Jason stayed the first few days to make sure that Wyatt and I were comfortable and well taken care of before returning home. He didn't like the idea of leaving me and Wyatt in an unfamiliar city so far from home. It was important for him to see that we were both safe and protected. He also had the chance to see what day-to-day life would be like for us at KKI. He was able to attend Wyatt's family meeting that outlined Wyatt's care plan for his stay at KKI. I wanted Jason to feel like he was as much a part of Wyatt's recovery as I was. Plus, I thought it was important for him to be able to tell Jay what was going on with Wyatt. Jay had begun to panic when we told him Wyatt was going to go back to the hospital. He was terrified that Wyatt had gotten sick again. We began to affectionately call KKI the exercise hospital. It was the best way for me to communicate what goes on during a rehab stay, and it made the hospital seem much less scary for Jay.

Wyatt's schedule was similar to his inpatient stay at Shriners, which made an easy transition for us both. He had a total of four hours of therapy each day, plus his scheduled therapeutic recreation time. I fell in love with the spine gym the minute I walked through the door. It wasn't the equipment. It was the people. Therapists, patients, and families all working beside one another and able to see and support others in the room. It felt much more like going to work out at the YMCA than a hospital therapy room.

The motto for the International Center for Spinal Cord Injury was "Hope through Motion," and I could feel hope welling up in my soul. The therapists were always smiling and always encouraging. It became normal to hear cheers shouted through the room when a new milestone was reached for a patient.

One of two attitudes tends to prevail in rehab. There are people who have accepted their injury and situation and are working hard to regain what was lost, and there are people who aren't ready for acceptance and are angry. We were blessed to be surrounded by patients and families who fell in the first category.

It was not by chance that we ended up at KKI at the same time as so many wonderful families. I am sure it was part of God's plan. Wyatt ended up having three other children under the age of four staying as inpatients with spinal cord injuries at the same time. Two of the children even had transverse myelitis like Wyatt. He instantly had playmates going through the same thing. He was too young to develop true friendships, but having therapy next to kids his own age had to make the situation feel normal to him, and I needed to meet other families. I needed the companionship more than Wyatt. At home, I had felt like I had been wandering through the desert, isolated and alone. No one I knew faced a similar storm. Having the opportunity to talk and spend time with other parents going through a pediatric spinal cord injury was invaluable.

Wyatt just smiled through his therapy. I don't think he realized that he could start crying and object. He was such a people pleaser. He was just born that way. All his therapist had to do was cheer and clap, and Wyatt would attempt whatever was asked of him, even if it was hard. It made the therapy process so much easier for me. I don't know if my heart could have handled Wyatt crying through every session. The few times he did get upset, I had to leave the room because I wanted to scoop him up and tell him he didn't have to keep working so hard. I would have done him a disservice if I had let him quit, so instead, I sat in another room and cried while his therapist pushed him through his tears.

One of my favorite parts of therapy was watching Wyatt "walk" on the treadmill. It wasn't really walking, but it was close enough for me. Wyatt used a piece of equipment called a LiteGait. It was a large metal frame with a harness attached to it, and it would suspend Wyatt over the treadmill with his feet touching for partial weight-bearing. He had a therapist working each leg, and one holding his hips still, and they would move his legs in a walking motion. His therapist made it look easy, but it wasn't. Their arms got an amazing work out as they moved Wyatt's legs in a normal walking pattern. It was incredible to watch, but the absolute best part was listening to a room full of patients and therapists singing *"The Ants Go Marching."* Even the teenage boys were singing! It made therapy fun.

Wyatt's first therapy session on the LiteGait was the morning after Jason left to return home. I hated that he had to miss it. I instantly realized how many firsts Jason was going to miss, and I did my best to document every moment to share with him.

Wyatt was also able to have therapy in the pool. The pools at KKI were state-of-the-art and the coolest thing I'd ever seen. The floors of the pools were adjustable, allowing a therapist to customize the pool depth depending on a patient's needs. It also made entry into the pools easy. The buoyancy of the water let therapists work on skills without the full force of gravity. Gravity is not a friend to those with a spinal cord injury, and movement was much easier beneath the surface of the water. The pools and the room were kept at a high temperature to keep patients comfortable and prevent muscle spasms. It felt like a sauna. It made me sleepy, and more than once I nodded off during one of Wyatt's sessions.

It's easy to paint a happy picture of therapy, but I don't want to lessen or minimize the work that was involved. I had grown up around sports. I ran track and cross country in high school and college and had worked for a minor league hockey team. I knew how athletes worked and trained, and these kids were tougher than any athlete I had ever seen. They weren't spending hours a day training to play in front of a cheering crowd and win a medal. They were using every ounce of energy they had day after day to simply learn to lift a finger.

It was humbling to watch. Being surrounded by children who were unable to breathe on their own or use their arms put everything in perspective. I was beyond blessed. I had been upset all along that Wyatt had lost the use of his legs, but I should have been celebrating what he could do. I marveled at the strength I saw in other parents. They were such an encouragement to me. For the first time since Wyatt's paralysis, I felt like I was part of a true community. The stories were different, but our aches were the same.

When the KKI trip began to come together, I knew my visions of an elaborate first birthday party were gone. The calendar did not lie, and time could not stand still. September 24th fell right in the middle of Wyatt's KKI stay. Birthday number one would be celebrated in a hospital far away from friends and family. It was a trivial thing to cry over, but I cried anyway. I don't know why the first birthday had become such a big deal, but I suddenly felt cheated out of a fancy cake, themed finger food, matching plates, and goody bags. I loved planning an Elmo party for Jay's first birthday and baking Minnie Mouse cupcakes when Austin turned one. I know Wyatt had no knowledge of dates. I could have easily thrown a big party once he returned home, but sometimes we lose our sense of reason when our emotions run high. I certainly did.

I spent my nights lying next to Wyatt's crib talking to God. In the quiet, I poured out my heart. I told Him everything. I had never been one to hide my feelings from God. He already knew my every thought so there was no point in keeping them from Him. I told God when I was sad and when I was angry. I told Him when I was lonely and felt forgotten, but most nights, I told Him I felt guilty. I felt guilty for being sad because, after all, my baby was alive. I felt guilty that my baby could breathe on his own and move his arms and fingers, because down the hall there were moms who couldn't say that. Just down the hall were moms listening to the sounds of machines breathing for their children and praying their children could be as healthy as Wyatt. There I was crying because my baby couldn't walk, and another mom simply wanted her baby to breathe.

There was no big epiphany or message from God in the midst of tears. My Father just held me until my crying was done, until I could see a reason to celebrate. Wyatt's first year didn't look like I had imagined. Nothing went as planned, but my baby was alive. His life was a gift, and I decided I would not spend the day mourning what could have been. I was going to celebrate the life that remained.

My mom sent a box of birthday goodies for Wyatt. I had hung Sesame Street decorations from the ceiling. There was a Happy Birthday banner taped across the door when I woke on the morning of his birthday. I couldn't wait to give Wyatt his presents. I managed to let him finish breakfast before I sat the first gift before him. I watched as his little hands struggled to rip the colorful paper. I made a small tear in the side of the paper and then watched as he tore open the paper to reveal a toy car.

I'm sure somewhere my dad was feeling a pain in his chest at the thought of his grandchild opening a birthday present before the cake had been cut. It was totally against the Wallis family tradition to open gifts at breakfast. My dad has been convinced since his own childhood that gifts were reserved for the end of the birthday, after candles had been blown out and cake had been eaten. He has always told me it's tradition, but nothing in Wyatt's first year had been traditional, so we opened presents first.

To my surprise, there was a special birthday party for Wyatt during therapy in the spine gym. His party was complete with gifts, cupcakes, party hats, and even a special smash cake just for him. There in the gym I stripped Wyatt down to his diaper, put a party hat on him, hooked a blue striped bib around his neck, and sat him down in front of his cake. His therapist supported his back as he sat smiling in front of this cake, and everyone in the gym sang Happy Birthday and watched as Wyatt plunged his hand into the white icing on the cake.

He had the biggest, cake-covered smile I had ever seen, and his eyes shone with complete and total joy. He didn't need a fancy themed party with coordinating invitations. He just needed to feel loved, and he did without question—and so did I. It was more special than anything I could have planned on my own. The backdrop of a hospital turned out to be the perfect setting to celebrate.

Wyatt had accomplished so much in his first year. He worked so hard each day to merely play with a toy or army crawl across the floor. I was so proud of all he had done, but I wanted more for him. I wanted to make life easier for him. When his OT mentioned that she was going to try to find a small wheelchair for Wyatt to try, my heart filled with excitement. There had been a time that the thought of my child in a wheelchair would have left me in a heap on the floor, but I had gotten past my fears. I wanted what was best for Wyatt, not what was most comfortable for me. After being at KKI, I saw a wheelchair as freedom and independence, and I wanted that for Wyatt.

A couple days after Wyatt's birthday, he was able to try a wheelchair for the first time. His OT Kaitlin found the smallest wheelchair in the hospital, but when she sat Wyatt in the chair, his arms couldn't reach the wheels. It was still too big for my little munchkin. Kaitlin decided to remove the seat cushion, and she found a thin gel pad to place on the seat. With the seat cushion removed, Wyatt could reach the wheels. Kaitlin buckled his seatbelt and wrapped a strap around his chest to keep him from falling over. She unlocked the brakes and placed Wyatt's hands on the wheel and showed him how to push.

Kaitlin grabbed a light-up stacking toy and walked across the gym. I stood beside her with my phone in hand, recording every second. She held the toy out and called Wyatt to her. I thought my heart might pound out of my chest. I had watched in delight as Jay and Austin took their first steps, and this was more than the equivalent for Wyatt. He reached down and put his hands on the wheels and made the smallest push, and then he did it again as Kaitlin continued to call him to her. Halfway to her, he got distracted and stopped to play with the gel pad he was sitting on. He wasn't nearly as impressed with his own achievement as everyone else in the room. Kaitlin called Wyatt again, and he continued to push to her. He stopped in front of her with outstretched arms, waiting to play with his toy.

He had done it. He had gotten from point "A" to point "B" on his own, and a whole new world of independence and exploration was opened up to Wyatt. I couldn't believe my eyes. I knew the ability to move around freely would change everything for Wyatt. It wasn't walking, but it was still a miracle. Immediately, I began texting the video to family, and then I uploaded the video to Wyatt's Facebook page. It seemed so surreal. Just months earlier, I was begging God for restoration to avoid a wheelchair, and suddenly I found myself in a room cheering and fighting back tears as my son made his first pushes across the floor. God had opened my eyes to the opportunities in front of Wyatt, and everything about my perspective changed. Life goes on even when healing is incomplete.

I shared the video of Wyatt's first time in a wheelchair on a "Good News" post on our local Fox affiliate's Facebook page. The comment with the most likes was supposed to be mentioned on the evening news. I thought it would be really neat if Wyatt's picture ended up in the news. I knew Jay would love to see it, but I never expected Wyatt's story to take off the way it did. Wyatt's story won the "Good News" feature, and before I knew it, there was a link to Wyatt's Facebook page to go along with the small news story. There were over a thousand new likes on his Facebook page, and my phone began chiming with message after message. I got messages from adult wheelchair users, parents of children in wheelchairs, and people who just thought he was cute. I even received a request from the Huffington Post asking if it was okay to share Wyatt's story.

It was exciting and scary all at the same time. I had no idea so many people would want to follow Wyatt. I didn't realize that his story seemed so incredible to other people. I knew he was an amazing little boy, but I was his mommy and completely biased. I know much of the response was simply the novelty of a bald-headed baby pushing a large chair that proportionately made Wyatt look even smaller than he was. I read message after message offering me encouragement, sending prayers, and telling me that Wyatt was an inspiration. The more the readership on his Facebook page grew, the more I felt an overwhelming responsibility to openly and honestly share our struggles, triumphs, and the source of our strength.

I wanted the hope of the gospel to be evident through the story I shared. Even when it was hard, I wanted what I wrote and shared to paint a picture of the goodness of the Father. I didn't want the world to see a picture of a baby in a wheelchair as a reason to believe that God wasn't good. I also didn't want to mistakenly lead anyone to believe that I had it all together or that somehow this life wasn't hard because I was a Christian. I was still a mess of emotions most of the time. It was still hard, and even in the midst of celebrating Wyatt's newfound freedom in a wheelchair, I felt like I had been kicked in the gut as newfound complications arose.

Wyatt got sick fast. Without warning, his temperature rapidly rose to over 104. He was shaking and sweating, and I was completely terrified. His little body felt like it was on fire. His doctors immediately suspected a urinary tract infection (UTI) was to blame, and a quick test revealed he had a raging UTI. He was immediately started on antibiotics and IV fluids to help flush the infection from his body. His nurses had trouble getting the IV started in his arm, and he had to be taken to the treatment room to have an IV placed in his head once again.

In a typical, healthy child, a UTI wouldn't be a cause for great concern, but Wyatt wasn't typical. I knew what this meant for him, and a short time later, I was told Wyatt needed to begin a catheterization program. It was the reality I most wanted to avoid. I knew paralysis affected Wyatt's bowel and bladder control, but since he was a baby, I had been able to pretend like it didn't. He was supposed to be in diapers, and I had hoped he would have enough recovery by the time he was older to not need them. I just tried not to think about it. His diapers were wet, so I just assumed that everything was working okay. It wasn't.

His doctors explained to me that although Wyatt's bladder was releasing urine, it likely wasn't able to empty fully, allowing old urine to sit in the bladder. This was probably what caused the UTI, and to prevent any additional UTIs and protect the kidneys, Wyatt needed to be catheterized every four hours. He had been scheduled to have a urodynamic study to examine his bladder and kidneys, but it had to be canceled due to the infection. It would have to be done once we returned home.

I wanted to sit in the corner and cry. I didn't want this for Wyatt, and I didn't feel confident in my own abilities to catheterize Wyatt. His nurse Erika came to teach me how to do the catheterization. She was so encouraging and positive that I'd be able to do everything at home on my own. It just all seemed so wrong and unfair to me, but there was no way around it. So I learned, and for once, I was thankful that Wyatt couldn't feel what was happening to him. He wouldn't even wake during his night time catheterizations. I let his nurses handle the night time shift since I knew once we returned home, I would no longer be able to sleep through the night.

The timing of it all was actually a blessing for me. I felt like I had been spoon fed little bits of information and new diagnoses along the way. I couldn't have handled the catheterization at the time Wyatt was initially diagnosed. I am convinced that it would have sent me over the edge, but by this time I had grown used to what Jason and I affectionately referred to as our "new normal." This was just one more hurdle in a line of many that we had grown used to jumping.

The KKI staff worked to equip me to care for Wyatt at home once we left the doors of the hospital. Recovery wouldn't have meant much if I was not able to continue his care at home, and I was shown a world of possibilities available to Wyatt. Wyatt was experiencing a physical rehabilitation, but I was experiencing an emotional one. During Wyatt's initial stay at Shriners, I wasn't ready for it. It was all too fresh. The wounds in my heart were still bleeding, and I wasn't ready to accept a life without a complete healing for Wyatt.

Time had given my broken heart an opportunity to heal, and I began to understand that life could be full and amazing even when it didn't look like a storybook. I would have told you that I believed that from the beginning, but I didn't know how to live it. I was doing my best to stay positive and keep a smile on my face, but inside I had been wading in a pool of mourning over lost hopes and dreams instead of diving into the depths of possibilities. I had been living life in the shallow end, and I realized that I didn't have to stay there. My eyes were opened to the possibilities before me.

God didn't make me or Wyatt or anyone for a life of simple existence. We were made to live and experience life to the fullest, whatever that may look like. I understood for the first time that living life to the fullest for me and Wyatt didn't have to look like everyone else's lives. I wasn't bound by anyone else's perceptions of normal any more than Wyatt was by his wheelchair. I found freedom the more I leaned into the Father. When I finally released the haze of comparison, the joys before me became clear. Within the walls of that hospital, I realized how little I actually needed to be happy. I had one drawer full of clothes and a chair to sleep on, and God showed me that it was enough. He was enough. My heart was content. My fulfillment came through relationships, not stuff.

I still count the friendships I formed with other parents as one of my greatest joys from KKI. I loved being able to fellowship and experience life together with other parents learning the same lessons I was learning. I don't think any of us really had a clue what we were doing. Each day was a new adventure or battle, and we all just did the best we could for our children.

Toward the end of Wyatt's stay, we took a therapeutic leave of absence (TLA) to the Baltimore waterfront with a few other patients and parents. We had become close to another patient named Bella and her mom Crystal. Bella also had TM and celebrated her third birthday at KKI a few days after Wyatt turned one. Bella was strong and beautiful and left a trail of glitter wherever she went. Wyatt loved to be around her. I think she must have reminded Wyatt of his own strong-willed sister at home.

The subway was across the street from the hospital, and since we didn't have a car with us, we were taking a subway ride to the waterfront. Bella was in her wheelchair, and I was pushing Wyatt in a special needs stroller. It was only the second time I had ever ridden on a subway, and I wasn't completely confident in what I was doing or where I was going. I don't think Crystal was any more confident than I was, but we felt a little strength in numbers. We figured if we were lost, at least we'd be lost together.

We successfully bought our tokens and read the map to figure out which direction we should be headed. We pushed Wyatt and Bella onto the subway and found a seat. We were feeling pretty good about ourselves until the subway took off. We had neglected to lock the brakes on Wyatt's stroller and Bella's wheelchair, and when the train took off, they rolled away. Crystal and I jumped up to grab them before they rolled to the other side of the car. We felt stupid, but we laughed hard and learned a valuable lesson. That split second of panic is etched in my brain, and I am still constantly checking to make sure Wyatt locks the brakes on his wheelchair.

I used a special needs stroller for Wyatt at KKI when he wasn't practicing in the wheelchair. He only used the wheelchair to roll from his room to therapy since there wasn't a seat cushion and his therapist didn't want to risk him developing a pressure sore. I was continuing to take videos of Wyatt in his wheelchair to send home to Jason. I was eagerly anticipating ordering Wyatt's his first wheelchair when we got home, but Jason didn't want to wait. The process of ordering a wheelchair can take up to six months, and Jason was worried Wyatt would lose all the independence he worked so hard to gain. He wanted Wyatt to have a wheelchair made especially for him, but he knew Wyatt needed something to fill in the gap.

I began asking and calling hospitals near home, but no one had anything small enough for Wyatt to borrow. I searched Craigslist and eBay hoping that I would be able to find something we could buy. I had already gotten lucky and found a special needs stroller on eBay. I was even able to have it delivered to the hospital to be serviced before we left. I felt like I was already batting a thousand.

Since children usually grow out of pediatric medical equipment long before the equipment is worn out, a lot of good pediatric equipment ends up for sale online. If you have patience and are persistent, you can often find inexpensive used medical equipment. After a week of repeated looking, I found the tiniest, neon green wheelchair for Wyatt. We won the auction for under $200 and had it shipped home, where it would be waiting on Wyatt.

At the beginning of Wyatt's stay, I thought five weeks sounded like such a long time, but time flew by quickly. Before I knew it, Jason, Jay, and Austin were headed to Baltimore to bring me and Wyatt home. It was such a bittersweet time. I had desperately missed Jason, Austin, and Jay, but I didn't want to leave. Wyatt had made so much progress, and I knew we couldn't replicate the same level of intensity at home. I was scared home would slow his recovery, but I wanted my family back together more than anything else.

CHAPTER 9

FAST FORWARD

Now to him who is able to do immeasurably more than all we
ask or imagine, according to his power that is at work within us.

~ Ephesians 3:20

WYATT GAINED SO MUCH STRENGTH during his stay at KKI, and it was unmistakably evident to us before we even made it home. We stopped to stay the night in a hotel halfway between home and Baltimore because we had spent the day together at the aquarium and were too tired to continue driving. The aquarium visit was a fun celebration of having our family reunited as well as an opportunity to make positive memories and take advantage of all the travel Wyatt's paralysis created. We like to find something fun for the entire family any time we travel out of town for medical treatment.

We stopped and grabbed some fast food for dinner to bring to the hotel before we checked in. In the middle of settling in for the evening, we sat Wyatt in the center of the bed with a plate of french fries. I had intended to put a few things away and set up Wyatt's travel crib before helping him eat since we didn't have a highchair for him, but he didn't wait for me. With one arm propped on a pillow, he grabbed a french fry off the plate and put it in his mouth. It was a wow moment, absolute visual proof of progress.

It wouldn't have looked like much to anyone else, but it was to us. Just five weeks earlier, Wyatt couldn't even come close to feeding himself without support. He needed to use both hands simply to hold himself up to keep from tumbling over. He was essentially stuck in the sitting position, but after five hard weeks of therapy, Wyatt was sitting on a soft, unstable surface and lifting his arm to feed himself. He wasn't standing or running across the room, but we cheered as if he were. Small victories lead to bigger ones, and even if the big ones never come, the small ones are worth celebrating.

Home was exciting. Wyatt's temporary wheelchair arrived, and it gave him new freedom. It was the tiniest little thing. It only came up to the bottom of my knee and was the perfect height to put him eye level with his classmates at school. It was a little heavy for him to push around on his own, but it gave him so much more freedom than being strapped in a stroller.

Wyatt's increased strength gave him the ability to explore and play more on his own. He learned to transition from a sitting position to his stomach, and he gained enough strength to do a true army crawl across the floor. There were moments when I didn't know if I should jump up and celebrate or sit on the floor and cry as I watched him drag his body across the floor. It took so much energy for him to get from one side of the room to the other. By the time he reached the toy he desired, he had to rest before he could play with it, but he was never deterred.

Fox Carolina, the news station that showed Wyatt's video during his stay at KKI, followed up with a full story on Wyatt after he returned home. It was the most precious story and focused on what Wyatt had accomplished, not what he had lost. It was important to me that the world didn't look at Wyatt with sad eyes. Wyatt wasn't sad. He was happy, enthusiastic, and thriving, and I wanted everyone to see that side of him.

I knew Wyatt would need a wheelchair built specifically for him. The one he was using did not provide nearly enough support to use for an extended period of time. I didn't realize how little I knew about wheelchairs until I began to research them. I thought a wheelchair was a wheelchair, but I was highly mistaken. Having a correct fit is especially important for those with paralysis who cannot feel if something is rubbing again them. The other major issue is the weight of a wheelchair. Wyatt was barely twenty pounds, and a lot of the pediatric wheelchairs were upwards of fifty pounds. Clearly the weight of a wheelchair will affect one's mobility.

God laid out a path that led to the perfect wheelchair to meet Wyatt's needs. I assure you that it wasn't a genius move on my part. When Wyatt's story aired on Fox Carolina, it was shared across the county. It led to a lot of new followers on Wyatt's Facebook page. One was the mother of another young child who was also a wheelchair user. Her son began pushing his own wheelchair well before his first birthday, and he was involved in WCMX, wheelchair motocross, which is an adaptive skateboarding sport.

She suggested that we look into a company called Box Wheelchairs. I did, and I was blown away by the chairs they were building. It was like going to look at a Ferrari after thinking that only sedans existed.

These chairs were a game changer. They were lightweight and durable, everything I wanted for Wyatt. At the time, the Box Wheelchairs did not process through insurance, but God made a way for the payment as well without any sacrifice by our family—because a much greater sacrifice had already been made.

Heather Gray and I had grown up together. We had known each other since elementary school, and our foundation in Jesus was built at the same church. I even accompanied her family on a memorable cruise when we were in middle school. We lost touch after high school, but thanks to Facebook and a class reunion, we were able to reconnect.

Heather's husband, Air Force Major David Gray, was killed in action in Afghanistan in 2012, leaving behind Heather and three beautiful children. She created Finish Strong Ministries to honor David's memory and to share the legacy he began. Heather contacted me through Facebook and said that Finish Strong wanted to support Wyatt and purchase his first wheelchair.

My heart was humbled and completely overwhelmed. I hate that I didn't get a chance to know Maj. Gray this side of heaven, but every day my son's life is better because of him and Heather's willingness to find beauty in brokenness and to make good from the bad.

While waiting for Wyatt's wheelchair to be built, we were able to get thorough testing done on Wyatt's bladder at Shriners Hospital in Greenville. The UTI he had at KKI wasn't a fluke thing. I had hope that the testing would allow us to quit catheterizing Wyatt, but I was living in a bit of a dream world.

Wyatt was diagnosed with a neurogenic bladder and a vesicoureteral reflux. His bladder was basically having spasms all the time, and the pressure in his bladder was so high that it was forcing urine back up to the kidneys. It was news that I didn't want to hear, but I knew we had to do anything and everything possible to protect his kidneys. We continued cathing Wyatt every four hours, and he started taking medicine to relax his bladder and prevent UTIs.

It definitely took some time to get adjusted to cathing him on a four-hour schedule. I suddenly began to look at life in four-hour increments. I cathed him at eight o'clock, twelve o'clock, and four o'clock. It wasn't the ideal schedule for sleeping, but it allowed me to drop Wyatt off at his half-day preschool and pick him up without a need to be cathed in between. The nights were certainly hard. I felt like I suddenly had an infant again and was unable to sleep through the night. Thankfully, I never had any trouble falling back asleep, and Wyatt typically slept through the whole catheterization at night.

Jason learned to cath Wyatt in case of an emergency, but it wasn't something he felt comfortable doing on a regular basis, not in the beginning, anyway. My mom and my sister both learned to cath Wyatt as well, which was essential in giving me and Jason a break from the kids to have a little time alone. Without their willingness to learn to care for Wyatt, Jason and I would never have been able to have a night away from the kids. I am convinced we would have both pulled all our hair out by now if we had no opportunities to get away and recharge.

We had hoped that the medication prescribed to Wyatt would have been enough to lower the pressure in his bladder, but unfortunately, it wasn't. He had to have Botox injections in his bladder, which paralyzes the bladder and prevents it from having spasms and creating pressure. Wyatt had to be put to sleep under general anesthesia for the injections, but it was a quick outpatient procedure with no recovery time needed. The Botox lasts for four to six months, and we follow up with testing and repeat the Botox when it wears off. I personally think moms of children who need Botox injections should get complimentary Botox injections for the wrinkles that all their children's medical issues create. I'm sure there has to be a little bit of medicine left in the syringe. It would make the process more enjoyable.

Wyatt's Box Wheelchair arrived at the end of February 2014, and it was everything we hoped it would be. It weighed only twenty pounds, and it was so much easier for Wyatt to push than the chair he had been using. He could go farther and longer in his chair because he wasn't exhausted. The weight also made it much easier for me to move the chair around. I didn't have to hurt my back getting it in and out of my van, and I could even pick the chair up with Wyatt buckled into it if necessary.

Wyatt's confidence blossomed in his new chair. He learned to go down ramps and pop wheelies. He was even able to push his chair through the grass with minimal assistance. We had to chase him around stores and restaurants because he refused to stay still. He wanted to explore everything and touch anything that was within reach. He didn't have any concept of safety and regularly attempted to give me a heart attack by trying to fall off curbs. I think he would willingly drop off the edge of the Grand Canyon if we let him. He had absolutely no fear in his chair.

His new chair created quite the scene wherever we went. I think it was partly due to the "Eat My Dust" license plate proudly displayed on the back and partly due to the fact that Wyatt looked so very young. His bald head made him look as much as six months younger than his actual age, and people were often caught off guard when they saw him pushing the chair on his own. I'm sure it was a rare sight. I think we heard it all, from "Oh, he's so cute" to "Oh, that's so sad." Neither response really made any sense to me. I was regularly asked if he was "born that way," and when I would explain what happened, I'd get the most pitiful looks. I never understood why some people thought it was somehow sadder because he wasn't formed that way in my womb.

The strangest comment I heard was at the mall when a lady walked up to me and said, "That little wheelchair is the best idea. I wish I would have thought about using a wheelchair when my daughter was little. It looks so much better than pushing them around in a stroller."

I had no idea how to even remotely begin to respond to that statement. I decided it was best to politely smile and nod my head. The wheelchair certainly was not a choice we wanted to make. The absurdness of the comment didn't even bother me. It made me recognize how little people actually pay attention to the words that are coming out of their mouths. After that statement, nothing really surprises me anymore.

Jay and Austin quickly caught on to the attention their little brother created, and they took great pride in pushing him around in public. I think Jay had a magic speed sensor that activated in his hand every time he grabbed the handle of Wyatt's chair. We couldn't get Jay to keep up with us when we were all walking together, but as soon as he started pushing Wyatt's chair, he would take off like he was in the middle of a speed walking championship.

Wyatt would laugh as the air rushed past his face, and that just encouraged Jay to go faster. More than once, I thought Jay was going to flip Wyatt out of his chair when he decided to make a sharp ninety-degree turn in the middle of a full-on run through the mall. I had to threaten Jay with punishment for continuing to run ahead with Wyatt.

The attention Wyatt generated was a little tough to get used to at first. It bothered Jason much more than it did me. I actually loved the chance to tell Wyatt's story. His chair had wheel covers that said "Finish Strong," and any time someone would ask about the chair, I would have the chance to tell them about Maj. Gray, his love for Jesus, and all Jesus had done for us. I wanted to tell Wyatt's story with hope, not sadness.

Jay thought his little brother was famous because he had been on the news, and he loved to talk to everyone about it. If anyone he didn't know ever mentioned Wyatt, Jay would stop to tell them that his brother had been on the news, and he would tell them how to find Wyatt on Facebook too. He especially loved to take Wyatt to school to show off to his classmates. I almost hated to bring Wyatt to any of Jay's school functions because I didn't want to take attention away from Jay. But Jay always wanted Wyatt there. He would beam with pride as he pushed Wyatt around his school, telling everyone that this was his little brother.

Jay's classmates each had a journal they wrote in as part of their Bible lessons. They had been talking about the miracles Jesus performed, and there was a space in the journal where the kids were asked to draw a picture of a miracle they had seen. I doubt I would have been able to come up with anything to draw at their age, but they had no trouble. Another parent sent me a picture of her son's journal, and he had drawn a picture of Wyatt in his wheelchair. When I asked

Jay about it, he told me his entire class had drawn a picture of Wyatt. A class full of second graders saw what so many adults didn't—that a baby in a wheelchair wasn't sad; it was a miracle.

We made several additional week-long trips back to KKI and Shriners in Philadelphia to monitor Wyatt's progress and make adjustments to this therapy. Wyatt also had the incredible opportunity to take part in a four-week summer rehab program at Shriners in Philadelphia. I had a bad habit of praying for good news. I still have it. It's really a selfish prayer that's all about me, but God is gracious and still hears it. When things weren't going my way and life seemed overwhelming, I found myself asking God to send me good news. I was really just asking God to send me a blessing to make me smile. I was looking for a light in the tunnel. God often reminded me that He is more than enough good news for me and I just needed to adjust my thinking. That being said, I'm convinced that the summer rehab program was an answer to one of my "I need some good news" prayers.

The program wasn't even on our radar. I had no idea it existed until I got a call out of the blue asking if Wyatt would like to participate. Absolutely, positively, the answer was yes. We cleared everything on our calendar for the month of July, and we loaded everyone up to spend four weeks of our summer in Philadelphia so Wyatt could participate in the Therastride program. It was perfect timing for us as a family since the kids were out of school. Jason's dad was able to help cover everything at our office, and Jason had to leave for only a few overnight trips during the month.

Therastride provides gait training on a body-weight supported treadmill that includes sophisticated computer software to monitor the patient's progress. The summer rehab program gave Wyatt an opportunity to have forty-five minutes each day on the Therastride treadmill and an additional thirty minutes working on gait training on the ground. Doctors and therapists hope that the gait training will help to rewire the pathways of the nerve impulses from the brain to muscles. That's just a really fancy way of saying we really hoped that Wyatt could get stronger and possibly take a step on his own.

Caroline, Wyatt's original PT at Shriners, moved shortly after his first stay in Philadelphia. Wyatt's new PT was Marci Bienkowski, and we fell in love with her instantly. She was great with Wyatt and helped him work hard every day, even when he was a little cranky. Marci didn't even seem to mind when Jay and Austin got out a little out hand in the middle of a therapy session. Wyatt had a little movement in his hip flexor muscle that allowed him to pull his leg up. If he was crawling or lying on the floor, his legs would pull up into a frog-legged position. We weren't sure if he had control over it voluntarily, but we hoped he could use that little bit of movement to generate a swing of his leg. Wyatt had absolutely no ability to lock his knees.

Wyatt wore his AFO braces to keep his feet and ankles straight and leg immobilizers to keep his knees locked in a straight position when he was working on gait training on the ground with Marci. She worked to teach him how to use his upper body to shift his weight in one direction to de-weight the opposite leg to make a swinging motion happen. It sounds as difficult as it was to communicate to a one-year-old. I didn't even understand how to make it happen. Thankfully, Marci had an abundant supply of patience.

There is some benefit to Wyatt never learning to walk before his paralysis. He doesn't have a natural instinct to walk normally, which benefits him when he's attempting to walk with leg immobilizer and braces. He has to lean back in a manner not conducive to a typical walking pattern, and he has been really good at figuring out what makes his body work.

Wyatt did a great job on the Therastride treadmill. He was happy, and he followed instructions well. He worked very hard, but it just didn't seem to translate into taking any intentional steps over ground. I think we were all a little disappointed until one morning when everything came together in one miraculous moment that will forever be seared into our memories. Marci rolled behind him on a stool and helped to support his upper body. Wyatt used the tops of her knees to lean on, and as he leaned in one direction, the opposite leg swung forward.

He did it, the first step.

Over a year of hard work, thousands of prayers, and an ocean of tears. It was all worth it. We cheered, and the sweetness of happy tears rolled down our checks. There was so much hope in that little leg swing. Wyatt knew he had done something good, but he didn't understand the significance of it. He just wanted the toy that his daddy was holding, and he was figuring out a way to get to it, like a typical one-year-old.

We took a little of our free time in Philadelphia to have family pictures made. Wyatt's OT, Dani, was also an amazing photographer. We met her on a beautiful summer evening for pictures at the Philadelphia Museum of Art. We wanted to get pictures of Wyatt in front of the famous *Rocky* steps leading up to the museum. It will forever be our dream for Wyatt to one day climb those seventy-two steps on his own, and we wanted to start getting pictures documenting his progress.

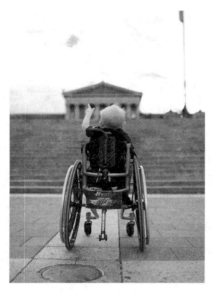

There are five landings from the bottom to top, and Jason wanted to use each section of sets as a goal, a milestone to reach, but Wyatt had to start at the bottom in his wheelchair. Jason and I both had an image in our minds of what we thought the picture would look like, but the actual photograph exceeded our expectations by a hundred times. Dani took pictures from behind Wyatt in his chair as he looked up to the top of the steps, and on his own, without any prompting, he pointed to the top like he knew what we were thinking. It was perfect, and it will forever be the perfect picture of our dreams for Wyatt, a picture that says more than an entire book of words can.

Before we had left home for Wyatt's summer rehab, Brian DeRoberts, an old high school friend, called me and said he wanted to have a fund-raising 5K race for Wyatt. Brian and I had run cross country and track together in high school, and he was now the head track and cross country coach at Woodmont High School in Piedmont, SC. He had followed Wyatt's story through my dad, who was coaching alongside him at Woodmont. He wanted to host an invitational race for high runners and include an open 5K race as a benefit for Wyatt, and just like that, the Fight Like Wyatt Invitational was born.

Brian did everything to put the race together. We basically just had to show up, and it all worked out wonderfully. There was a home football game at Woodmont High School the night before the race, and Brian made arrangements for Wyatt to lead the team onto the field. I can't tell you how excited Jay and Wyatt were at the football game. The crowd, the tunnel, the band. They were in amazement of the sights and sounds. It was a complete sensory experience for them. Fox Carolina even came to the football game and the race to do a follow-up story on Wyatt. It was perfect, and it was like a celebration for us.

I know I'm biased because I'm his mom, but Wyatt's fight is worth celebrating. It isn't the end result that counts, whether he walks or whether he doesn't. It is the beauty in the battle. The effort given. The smiles through pain. The endurance. The refusing to surrender when everything around you tells you to give up. It all matters. The journey counts because it's in the journey that we discover who we are following.

> *"My sheep listen to my voice; I know them, and they follow me."*
> ~ John 10:27

CHAPTER 10

FAITH LIKE A CHILD

And he said: "Truly I tell you, unless you change and become like little children, you will never enter the kingdom of heaven."

~ Matthew 18:3

NOT LONG AGO, I HAD to take Jay in for an eye exam. He was holding books too close to his nose and monitoring the steps on his Fitbit with his wrist an inch from his face. I repeatedly asked him if he had trouble seeing. He answered me like a snappy nine-year-old. No, he didn't have trouble seeing. He just liked to hold things close to his face. Of course you do, son, how silly of mom to think you had a problem. I ignored it for a while, but my father-in-law noticed too. He was concerned. So I made an appointment at the optometrist for Jay to get a full eye exam.

Jay wasn't excited about the idea until he realized it meant an early dismissal from school. Once missing school was mentioned, he desperately needed the exam and couldn't wait for the day to arrive. When I arrived to pick him up from school, the office called his classroom and asked his teacher to send him to the office for dismissal.

His teacher asked if I could wait a few minutes longer because the class had just started their weekly spelling test. I was uncharacteristically early and had more than enough time to wait. I laughed as I sat down on the long bench in the hallway because I knew the first words that were going to come out of Jay's mouth.

I heard the rolling of his book bag and the stomping of his boots coming down the hall, and I stood as he opened the security door to leave. He wasn't even through the door when I saw him shaking his head, and there it was. "Five minutes?" he said with a face-splitting smile. "You couldn't have been five minutes earlier, could you?"

We laughed as we made our way to the car. He was less than confident in his spelling test and was giving thanks for the dropping of the lowest test grade each quarter. The car ride to the optometrist was spent discussing his dislike for the spelling words on his test and specifically the word "frothy." He didn't believe it was a real word, and after I explained the definition, he still didn't believe he would ever have to use or spell the word in real life. He found it ridiculous. I told him that he might want to be a barista one day, and he'd need to know how to spell it. He was less than amused. I don't think he had any future plans involving Starbucks.

At the optometrist's office, I checked Jay in with the receptionist, and we found a couple of chairs together in the waiting area. I felt like I should have been doing something else, like something was missing. Jay and I sat together and just talked, and I realized how much easier doctor's offices are with a nine-year-old. Waiting rooms were typically not fun for me. They were normally places of exhaustion as I attempted to chase Wyatt and Austin and keep them entertained, but this was nice. Sitting, talking, and waiting with my oldest was relaxing.

I realized how little one-on-one time I actually had with Jay anymore. He was my sidekick when he was little. I took him everywhere with me, and he basked in the attention of being an only child. But now, my attention was divided by three, and we didn't often have the opportunity to spend time by ourselves. Jay's one-on-one time was normally reserved for his dad or his pop on tractors and trucks. I listened to him talk as we waited, astounded at the young man he had become. He had grown up overnight, and he relished the chance to take part in adult conversation.

When the nurse called his name, he jumped to his feet, and I followed him back to a room and sat in the corner while his eyes were examined. He told me he wasn't nervous, but he was, and I could tell. He is his father's son, and they both get silly when they get nervous. They think they are hilarious even if no one else does. They crack jokes about everything. I find the trait rather endearing in them both, even if it can be a little embarrassing for me at times. Laughter makes the hard things easier.

The nurse explained to Jay that she was going to put a few drops in his eyes, and he would need to sit in the dark for a few minutes while the drops dilated his eyes. She told him the drops wouldn't hurt at all, and he believed her. He looked up toward the ceiling and waited for her to put the drops in. As soon as the first drop hit his eye, he yelled out and reached up to cover his face.

"I don't know who told you those drops don't hurt, but they lied," he informed the nurse.

I shouldn't have laughed, but I did. He was so serious. He was fine ten seconds later, and we sat in a dark room while we waited for the doctor to come in and complete the examination. Jay read all the letters and answered all the questions. I expected him to need glasses, but the doctor said his eye sight was great. His eyes were just a little sensitive to light. Jay stood up from the examination chair and with both fists closed, he threw his arms into the air like he had just won the Daytona 500, like he was ready for someone to shower him with a freshly popped bottle of champagne.

"Yes!" he exclaimed. "I'm still the only one in the family without a medical history!"

I laughed out loud. I couldn't believe those words came out of his mouth. The doctor looked over at me a little shocked.

"Do you have a big medical history in your family?" she asked.

"You could say that," I answered. I didn't have hours of time to explain, so I left it at that.

Sometimes I forget how much Jay and Austin have been through. What nine-year-old thinks about a medical history? One who has watched his mom and dad go through serious surgeries. One who has spent countless hours sitting in hospitals waiting for his brother to finish therapy, and one who has seen his sister given a diagnosis of her own. Doctors, therapies, and hospital are normal for him. He's seen the mountains of paperwork and list of medicines that go along with each new appointment.

Siblings are often the forgotten warriors in a special needs family. Their battles don't take center stage, but they are fighting. They are battling with fears and emotions they can't control. They watch as their sibling struggles. They don't understand why Mommy and

Daddy aren't home. They're jealous of the toys, cards, and balloons showered upon their special needs sibling, and they get jealous when they miss out on the things their friends enjoy. It is not an easy road.

Anytime something difficult happens to a child, someone throws out the word *resilient*. *Don't worry. Kids are resilient. They'll be fine.* I've heard those words so much. Kids ARE resilient. Those words are true. I believe that with all my heart, but don't think for one second that kids aren't shaped by the tragedies that touch them. Jay and Austin are different because Wyatt is paralyzed.

Our lives stopped when Wyatt became paralyzed. Sports, friends, vacations, school, *everything* took a back seat to Wyatt's rehabilitation. It wasn't fair, but there was no other way. Wyatt's health couldn't wait. Jason and I struggled to balance Wyatt's needs, our family business, care for Jason's mom as her Alzheimer's progressed, and take care of Jay and Austin, and there simply wasn't enough of us to go around. My heart felt like it was constantly torn in pieces. No matter who I was caring for, someone was missing out.

I often felt guilty, and I worried Jay and Austin would be filled with resentment as they grew. I didn't ever want them to resent Wyatt and the attention he received, but most of all, I didn't want either of them to develop a resentment for God. They know Wyatt has no control over his health, but they know that God does. I don't want them growing up angry because God didn't fix it. They both prayed for their little brother to be healed. They still do, and they are still waiting for it to happen. It's hard to answer all their "why" questions when I don't know the reasons myself.

So I tell them the truth. I tell them that I don't know the reason Wyatt is paralyzed, but I know God will make good out of it. I tell them both that God has an amazing plan for their lives, and He is going to use everything they are going through to make them better people. I remind them how much God loves them. I don't want them to ignore the hard and the hurt, but I don't want them to live in it either. I want to teach them to find the rainbows in the storms. I want them to dance in the rain instead of hiding from it. I want them to see the lessons learned, and I try to point out when I see the bad turned to good.

Jay's second grade school year was particularly tough for him. Jason and I were away with Wyatt a lot, and school just couldn't be a priority. I'm sure there are moms cringing at those words, but sometimes the biggest education happens outside the classroom. We were in survival mode as a family, and we honestly did the bare minimum for Jay to get by. It was only second grade, and I wasn't worried about bad grades. I only wanted him to make it to the third grade. There were no big goals.

Jay didn't worry about it either until awards day. He sat through the end of year awards ceremony and watched as his friends were called up one by one to receive awards. He was the only student in his class who didn't make the honor roll, and it broke his heart. He tried to hide his tears, but I could see them. He was devastated, and it wasn't his fault. It was mine, and I sat in the audience wishing I had kept him home from school. Then he wouldn't have had to feel the hurt of being left out, but that hurt turned into a bigger motivator than I could have ever imagined.

Jay remembered what it felt like to miss out, and the little boy who didn't care about school suddenly did. He wanted to do well, and it was such a blessing. The next two years, Jay made the honor roll and earned the "Most Improved" award from his teachers. The biggest improvements he made weren't in his academic ability. They were in his character, and I couldn't have been prouder of him. The tears from second grade were replaced with cheers for a job well done and big hugs from his little brother and sister who were getting to see the value in hard work.

Austin is only seventeen months older than Wyatt. She was only two when Wyatt got sick, and she had no idea why Jason and I were suddenly absent. There was no way to make her understand the situation. Wyatt spent twelve weeks in the hospital the year following his diagnosis. Plus, he had an additional four weeks of outpatient therapy in Philadelphia. Jason and I were gone a lot, and Austin began to develop serious separation anxiety.

When we were home, she became glued to my leg. She couldn't be in a room by herself, and she wanted to be close enough to touch someone at all times. She needed that security, and I watched as Jay became her security blanket instead of me. Jay was the one constant in her life. As she bounced around from aunts to grandparents, Jay followed her, and she trusted he would always keep her safe.

I didn't realize how strong their bond had become until a storm developed one night. The first loud crack of thunder was followed by the pitter patter of her little feet running across the floor. Austin was in a dead sprint, and as I knelt down to hold her, she ran by me. She didn't want me. She wanted Jay, and he opened his arms as she ran toward him. He helped her climb on the couch, and he sat next to her under the blanket until the storm passed. Their relationship is beautiful, and I know it is stronger than anything I could have imagined. The hard times have knit their hearts together.

Austin and I recently ran to the store to grab a few things before dinner. Running out of milk creates big problems in our house, and I couldn't wait until morning to grab a new gallon. We hadn't decided yet what we would eat for dinner, and I was hoping a quick and easy idea would hit me at the grocery store. Before we arrived, from the back of my van, Austin asked if I could call Jay and ask him to make her scrambled eggs for dinner.

Scrambled eggs had become our quick and easy go-to dinner. I'd cut up some fruit to throw on the kids' plates too, and I'd feel like I was giving them a meal with some decent nutritional value. Plus, the kids loved eggs, and even better is that Jay learned to cook them himself. He and his pop would spend their Saturdays making giant breakfasts together with eggs, bacon, sausage, and biscuits. It was Cracker Barrel at home, and Jay loved to help.

Jay had been begging to cook eggs himself, but I fought him for a while, terrified he'd set the house on fire or burn his arm off being careless. I finally gave in and let him cook on his own. I watched from the corner of the kitchen as he carefully pushed the eggs around the skillet until they turned a buttery yellow. He sprinkled shredded cheese on the top and portioned them out on individual plates. He was so proud of himself. My nine-year-old could help cook dinner. (His clean-up leaves a little to be desired, but we'll work on that.)

When I heard Austin's voice asking for eggs from the back seat, I quickly grabbed my cell and called Jason's phone.

"Hey, Mom," Jay said as he answered.

"Austin wants you to make scrambled eggs for dinner. Can you do that for us?" I asked.

"Of course. Just call me when you leave the store, and I'll have them ready," he said.

"Great! I'll call you when we're leaving. Thanks so much," I said as I hung up.

Austin pouted. "I wanted you to ask Jay to make my eggs, not Daddy," she said.

"Sweetie, I did ask Jay to make your eggs. He answered the phone," I informed her.

"Oh," she said. "Jay's going to make such a good daddy when he grows up."

My heart just melted. I don't think there are any sweeter words a five-year-old could utter about her big brother. She was absolutely right. In the midst of all our family's struggles, Jay was learning how to be a caregiver. It was more than just being a helper and involving himself in physical tasks. Jay was learning how to care for someone else's heart. He was learning to love and encourage, and his little sister saw it.

Austin and Wyatt have developed their own special bond. It's more love-hate than Jay and Austin's relationship. Their close ages have created a little toggle switch in their relationship, and they alternate between best friends forever or mortal enemies, depending on the time of day and who is controlling the television. There is no in between with the two of them.

Austin is Wyatt's constant companion. She's normally in tow at all his appointments. It's still easy to pull her out of school for doctor's appointments and out of town therapies, and she provides a constant distraction for Wyatt during long waits. It's not unusual for someone to stop and ask me if the two of them are twins. Walking beside Wyatt in his wheelchair, Austin is eye-to-eye with him, and their resemblance to one another is unmistakable. My heart aches when I think that before long she will tower over him from his chair, and he will have to look up to her. For now, they are face-to-face and discovering the world together.

They have quite the little medical vocabulary between the two of them. One day on the way home from the doctor, they'd had enough of each other.

"Eczema, eczema, eczema!" Wyatt yelled at the top of his lungs.

"Mom, Mom, Mom!" Austin howled back. "Wyatt is saying *eczema,* and he doesn't even have it. I have eczema, and he's not allowed to say it."

I probably should have stopped the little exchange, but I knew that no matter how I handled it, one of them would be crying the rest of the way home. It wasn't a shining parenting moment, but I told Austin to just say something back that Wyatt had.

"Transverse myelitis!" she screamed.

"Eczema!" Wyatt shouted back.

For five minutes this back and forth exchange occurred between the two of them—until they both started laughing. I couldn't decide if I found the little exchange funny or sad. Three and five-year-olds shouldn't know what those words mean, but mine do. I can't change that, but I can always remind them that they aren't defined by the labels of this world, medical or otherwise.

Austin was diagnosed with celiac disease last fall, and I feel awful that Jason and I didn't catch it sooner. It's an autoimmune disorder that damages the lining of the intestines and causes other issues when she ingests gluten. We thought Austin was just whiney or acting out to get a little more attention. She always seemed to complain her stomach hurt whenever our full attention was on Wyatt or when it was time to go bed. In the middle of therapy or when I was working with him at home, she would try to climb up into my lap and tell me her belly was hurting. I'd lay her on the couch and tell her to rest, and then it would miraculously feel better when it was time to play.

She got progressively worse after school started. I was poisoning her with wheat and didn't know it. She was eating pancakes for breakfast, sandwiches for lunch, and spaghetti for dinner. Her diet was destroying her, and I was oblivious to it. After getting sent home from school multiple times, we knew something was really wrong. One evening Jason asked her if she didn't feel good, and her response pierced my heart.

"I don't ever feel good anymore, Daddy," she said.

I felt like I should have been wearing a t-shirt that said "World's Worst Mom." She had been hurting so badly that she never felt good, and I missed it completely. When Jason had his stomach problems, I spent a lot of time online trying to play doctor and searching for a reason for his pain. I learned more about stomach conditions than I ever cared to know. Now, standing in my bedroom, I finally put two and two together. Austin wasn't growing much. Her stomach was always hurting. She had eczema, and we already had one child with an autoimmune disorder. I searched the Internet for information on celiac disease, and the more I read, the more I was convinced she was suffering from it.

I made her an appointment with her pediatrician the next day. We had to get a stool sample to check for parasites and bloodwork to look for celiac disease. She was not nearly as laid back as Wyatt about the doctors, and it took the help of several people holding her down to get a single vial of blood. I'm not sure if Austin or I cried more. She was not made for pain, and my heart couldn't stand her tears.

A week later her doctor confirmed that she had elevated markers for an autoimmune disorder. We were referred to a pediatric gastroenterologist, one of the few specialists Wyatt had never seen. A biopsy of her small intestines confirmed her diagnosis, and we eliminated all wheat and gluten from her diet. It's not easy to do when life is busy, but Austin is so much happier and healthier than she used to be. She is growing and smiling, and she understands what she needs to do to keep herself healthy. She is a rule follower and wouldn't eat a plate of chocolate chip cookies if you placed them in front of her. She remembers what it felt like to hurt, and she's not going to do anything she knows will hurt her. The memory of her pain protects her from doing anything that would hurt her body. I can assure you I will use that analogy in at least one speech during her teenage years.

For the last three years, our big family vacation has been spent in Philadelphia for Wyatt to have physical therapy at Shriners. For a month each summer, we have made the Ronald McDonald House our home. It sounds glamorous, I know. There hasn't been a fancy beach trip or big Disney World extravaganza, but you wouldn't have known that by our kids' excitement level. They think the RMH is the best hotel on earth. There are playrooms, movie theaters, and a home-cooked meal every night. It is a real home, and I have fallen in love with the community it creates.

The RMH does more than keep our family together during treatments. It's a refuge from the medical world and a place to connect with other families fighting similar battles. We live side-by-side with families from different races, cultures, and religions. There are children fighting cancer, missing limbs, using wheelchairs, and some unable to breathe on their own, and Jay, Austin, and Wyatt have played alongside them all. They've learned to see people as they should, simply as people. They don't see race or disability. They see value in everyone they meet, and they've learned that play is a universal language.

I've watched them build Lego towers with children who don't speak a word of English, and they figure it out. Laughter is the same in every language. I've watched them adapt games for children who are unable to move. I've seen them pass game pieces to the foot of a child who had no use of his arms. They are learning what love and acceptance looks like, and I could have never taught them as much on my own. They aren't scared of people who are different because they focus on what is the same.

I wish I could wipe away all the pain my children have felt, but I don't ever want them to lose the lessons they have learned from it. They have so much compassion in their hearts. They have learned kindness and gentleness. They've learned to celebrate others' successes. They have learned the value of life. They are different because life has been hard. God didn't take away their hard, but He gave them an opportunity to grow into the most incredible young people. They are being refined in the fire, and I can't believe that I get to be part of that process.

When I began the process of putting our story into words, one of my biggest fears was writing a story that left Jay and Austin out. They are a part of this story, and I want them to always know how much I love them. They are so much more than Wyatt's big brother and sister.

I want them to always have my words, from my heart, written just for them. May they never doubt their mommy's love for them.

Dear Jay and Austin,

You two are amazing in every way. I know it's been hard watching Wyatt get sick and sitting through all of those doctors' appointments and therapies. You've made so many sacrifices to help make your little brother's life better. I know it doesn't seem fair, but I promise it's making you both into the most incredible people. While your friends have been working to improve their soccer skills or perfecting the ballerina twirl, you have been developing character.

Jay, you are an old soul, wise beyond your years. You are a protector at heart, and you do everything you can to keep Austin and Wyatt safe. I didn't teach that. It's who God made you to be. Before the beginning of time, God knew you, and He's using all the suffering you have had to watch to mold you into the most remarkable young man I've ever met. You are so hard on yourself. Don't be. I want you to always remember to see yourself as God sees you. You are a child of the King.

The heart you have for God blows me away, and it is evident to anyone who knows you. Your little brother and sister look up to you so much. You are their hero, and I couldn't ask for a better role model for their little eyes. They are blessed to have you as their big brother.

Austin, you are a princess, creative, strong-willed, and uniquely your own in every way. You bring sparkle, glitter, and a closet full of pink into our world. You do life at your own pace and aren't swayed by anyone else's opinions. You make us stop to see all the colors of the rainbow, beautiful individually and dazzling together. You are Wyatt's BFF, his partner in crime. You challenge him. You push him, and sometimes you even battle him. You've never once seen him as less or different. You have a soul that loves to celebrate, no matter how small the achievement, and I can't wait to see how God is going to use that trait.

I love every second of being your mom. Slow down, you two! You are growing up way too fast, and I'm trying my hardest to hold onto every moment. I don't want you to ever leave, but I can't wait to watch you spread your wings. You were made to do more than fly. You will soar, my loves. Soar high.

Love You Always,

Mommy

CHAPTER 11

WHAT GOD HAS JOINED

Though one may be overpowered, two can defend themselves.
A cord of three strands is not quickly broken.

~ Ecclesiastes 4:12

I BOUGHT A NEW BIBLE a couple of months ago. I had been using the same Bible since college. It was precious to me. It was burgundy leather and had my maiden name stamped in gold in the bottom right-hand corner, and it was full of all my notes. My heart was written in the margins. Colored pens and markers highlighted my favorite passages. Flowers were doodled on the corners of tattered pages. It was a record of a love affair with my Savior, and I wanted to use it forever. But it ended at Hebrews.

Age got the best of my Bible, and James through Revelation fell out. I carried it around for a while, constantly shoving the missing books back into the cover and hoping they wouldn't fall out as I walked into church. I looked into getting it rebound, but I never followed through with it. I finally went to the bookstore to purchase a new Bible, and I discovered the Beautiful Word Bible. It is glorious.

It's an NIV version of the Bible with beautiful—hence the name—illustrations of Bible verses. It is completely feminine and girly, and I absolutely fell in love with it. I even got my name stamped in gold—my married name.

Jason had been in Philadelphia with Wyatt for several weeks when I bought the Bible, but I couldn't wait to show him. Patience is not a virtue that shines through when I buy new things. Telling Jason about the Bible didn't seem like it was quite enough. He needed to see it with his own eyes to understand how perfect it was. So I took a picture and sent him a text message about my perfect new Bible.

"Look. I got a new Bible. I love it. It's beautiful, and it has my last name on it," I texted under a picture of my Bible.

"I say the same thing about you," he texted back.

He seriously typed that. I melted, and he officially got a pass for at least a year on any less-than-brilliant comments that may come out of his mouth. We're thirteen years in, and he still makes my heart flutter and knees weak.

I've made a zillion mistakes in this life, but picking Jason wasn't one of them. We met at the church where I grew up. It's probably a more accurate description to say we met through the church. Jason joined the church while I was away at college and began attending my Sunday school class, but we had never officially met. I knew who he was, but I don't think I really even knew his name. One Easter Sunday when I was home, I wore a gray dress with what Jason still says was an inappropriately high slit. I don't think the slit was that high, but I'm certain I was wearing a dress that I wouldn't let my daughter out of the house in. Whatever the dress looked like, it caught Jason's eye.

I was working for a minor league hockey team at the time, and Jason found himself at a hockey game later that week with a group of people from our church. Unbeknownst to Jason, the group included my sister Amanda. At some point in the evening, the topic of my dress was discussed. I don't know the exact words that were said, but after Jason was introduced to my sister who was sitting behind him, he felt like he had to ask me out to dinner. If I would've worn pants that Easter Sunday, we might not ever have gotten together. Proof that God can turn our bad decisions into good.

Jason was the only boy who ever loved me, and I'm still not sure why. He's treated me like a princess since the day he opened my car door on our first date. He was the one for me. I never once questioned that. We were married in December surrounded by Christmas trees and poinsettias. Jason cried through the ceremony, and we pledged to love one another for a lifetime, for better or for worse, in sickness and in health.

We didn't know what we were getting into. We just knew we were better together. We still are. The life we're living today doesn't look like the one we imagined all those years ago as we placed rings on each other's fingers, but I still feel like I'm getting to live out my fairy tale dreams. I just haven't gotten to the ever-after part yet. We're just living in the hard part that makes the ending feel so much sweeter.

I could not have survived the last five years without Jason by my side. I am simply not strong enough. He has been my rock, the one to pick me up on days when I felt like throwing in the towel. I can't even begin to tell you how much my love for him has grown as I've watched him develop over the last three years. In many ways, I think this has been harder on him than me. He's supposed to be the leader and the protector of the family, and he can't do anything to make it better. He can't make Wyatt better. Jason is a fixer, a problem solver, and the inability to fix our situation felt crushing.

He has had to stretch so much farther out of his comfort zone than I have. He let me have tunnel vision and allowed me to focus all my energy on Wyatt. When I stayed in the hospital with him, Jason was home being both Mommy and Daddy to Jay and Austin. He took them to school, made lunches, cleaned the house, did laundry, helped with homework, and fixed dinner. He did it all, and he was never once resentful or bitter about carrying a double load. He became more appreciative and worked harder to help when I came home.

In the last year, he's grown comfortable catheterizing Wyatt. It was the one thing he didn't want to have to do. It just hurt his heart too much, but he knew I needed help. And he needed to be able to stay with Wyatt for extended periods of time. Two months ago, we switched places. I left Jason and Wyatt in Philadelphia for therapy for three weeks to be home with Jay and Austin. Three years ago, that seemed unfathomable.

I had been warned by social workers that the stress of a special needs child can wreak havoc on a marriage. The grief, the worry, the blame, the guilt, the financial burden can all become too much when you multiply it by two imperfect hearts. But instead of tearing us apart, this battle has made us stronger. God brought us both to the point where we had to release control of the lives we were living and give it all to Him. This pressure cooker we have been living in has not melted us.

"Yet you, Lord, are our Father. We are the clay; you are the potter; we are all the work of your hand."

~Isaiah 64:8

I like the idea of being like clay. The possibility of becoming anything. We're just a heap of potential lying on the potter's wheel. Before clay is fired, it's soft, moldable, and able to be shaped by whatever it touches. The hands of the potter meticulously form it with intent and purpose. Its beauty is evident from the moment it is created, but its beauty doesn't make it useful. Its usefulness doesn't develop until it's put in the kiln. The fire is what has the power. The firing process changes the clay into a new substance. The clay becomes ceramic in the fire, and it is hard and unchangeable. The firing process gives the clay its distinct purpose. It changes it from something of only beauty to something of use. Its purpose is defined in the fire.

I don't like the fire, but I like what it turns me into, what it turns my marriage into. I want to have a purpose, and I want to be useful. I want to hold my shape no matter what comes against me, and I want my marriage to do the same. I don't want my marriage to turn to a big pile of mush every time the weight of this world comes upon us. Bad stuff is going to happen, but God has shaped me for a purpose. The fire is not comfortable, but if God doesn't pull me from it, He is going to use it to change me into a new substance, one that can withstand more than I could ever imagine.

The stresses of Wyatt's paralysis have not been easy on our marriage. It's hard work, but it's worthwhile work. Making our marriage a priority brings us close to God and each other, which in turn makes us better parents and better people. I will never be a marriage expert. There are probably thousands of marriage counselors who would tell us that we're doing it wrong, but it's what works for us.

Jason and I talk about everything. If you want to tell me something but don't want me to tell Jason, please don't tell me. If you do,

I'm going to tell Jason. It's that simple. I tell him everything, and I don't make any apologies for being that way. Communication has been the biggest key to weathering our storm. We talk about the good and the bad, when we're happy and sad. There have been so many tears as we've tried to process together everything that Wyatt has gone through. We were honest when we were angry and upset.

Jason has always dealt with problems head on. When we were dating and newly married, it drove me crazy. We'd have to sit down and discuss issues that may or may not be a problem ten years from now. If there was something he was unwilling to waver on, he told me immediately. There was no hiding it and no surprise down the road. We weren't even engaged yet when Jason told me that if he had a son, he wanted the boy to be named after him. As in, if you're not okay with this, we need to end this relationship now. He was completely serious, and Jay is a Jr., in case you're wondering.

I love to talk. I've been accused more than once of not having an internal thought. Jason regularly informs me that he doesn't need to know what I had for lunch. But I would rather skip over the things that bring conflict. I don't want to talk about the things that hurt, but Jason makes me. And he's been right all along. I know where he stands, and if I find myself wondering, I ask him. It's made it easier for me to make big decisions when he's not close by because I already know the desire of his heart before a crisis ever arises.

From the beginning, God's design for marriage has been oneness, for two to become one flesh. You can't have oneness if you don't communicate. Marriage doesn't instantly make your spouse a mind reader. If your heart is broken, you have to tell your spouse. If you're exhausted and overwhelmed, you have to share it. If you need help, ask for it. A burden shared is a burden lifted. Jason doesn't know that I'm about to crack unless I tell him, and I can't get mad if I don't tell and he doesn't figure it out.

We try not to wallow in self-pity. We want to find a way to always be thankful even in the bad stuff, but some days it's too hard. The doubt creeps in and we lose sight of the truth, and a woe-is-me mentality takes over. We have been blessed not to find ourselves in the pit of despair at the same time. If I had a bad day, Jason had a good one, and vice versa.

Jason and I have learned to extend grace to one another in this season. Most days, I need buckets of it. No matter how hard we try not to, sometimes we lose it. We get snappy and someone yells when they shouldn't, and then grace shows up. And we let it go and we put away the blame. If we didn't, we could spend hours arguing over garbage that needs to be taken out. It's not worth it. Let the other person be wrong sometimes. I'm not condoning an abusive relationship by any means, but sometime when the stress is piling on, we say things we shouldn't. Instead of yelling back or pointing out the other's mistake, we walk away.

We find a way to laugh together. I think you have to have a sense of humor in the middle of the messes of life. Jason and I laugh about the dumbest stuff, but it makes life so much more fun. Our kids have watched us try to make the other person laugh when they're having a bad day, and they've learned to do it as well. We tell cheesy jokes, and we make up corny songs. Laughter makes us enjoy each other's company. It makes life fun, and it provides a break from reality.

Our biggest marriage struggle in the midst of all the chaos has been to carve out time alone, away from the kids and all of life's demands. Jason and I need to be together. We don't need fancy dinners and exotic vacations; we just need a couple hours alone after we put the kids to bed, just to be in each other's presence. We are so blessed to have parents close by who love to watch their grandchildren and give us a break as well. When we make our relationship a priority, we are better at everything else. We are refreshed, recharged, and renewed, and we can fulfill the purpose God designed us for.

I could whisper into Jason's ear a million times how amazing I think he is, but it does more for him and our marriage when I tell others how incredible he is. Instead of griping to a friend when he makes a mistake, I choose to share praise instead of fault. The more I brag about him, the harder he works to be the man I know he is. My words to him are my public thank you for being everything that I need.

Dear Jason,

I can't believe I get to do this life with you. I'm the luckiest girl in the world, and I don't take this life I share with you for granted, not for a second. You are my best friend, the one I want to hold hands with and wake up next to every morning. I love being your wife and being the bearer of your name. It is one of my life's greatest honors, and I've never once regretted my decision to say *I do* to you. I never thought I would find someone who loves me as much as you do. You make me feel beautiful and special every minute of every day. Thank you for loving me big.

I know your heart aches because our life doesn't look like the one you always planned for us. It's been harder and everything has taken longer than you imagined. Don't be hard on yourself. You are amazing. Every decision you make is intentional and rooted in making life better for our family. I know that. I wish you could see yourself through my eyes. If you could, all your doubts and worries would be wiped away. Everything I need, I have in you.

You are the most incredible father. I know you won't believe me and there are a thousand things you wish you could do differently, but God made you to be exactly who Jay, Austin, and Wyatt need. They need you specifically to guide them through this life. You are raising them to be brave, independent, and bold, because that's who you are. They think you would conquer the world for them, and you would.

I don't thank you enough for the way you lead our family and hold us together. You never give up on anything. We could have broken when Wyatt got sick. It could have been a reason to just throw in the towel and say everything is too hard. But we didn't. You didn't. It made you love me more because it drew you closer to the One who formed you. This fire that we've been in has changed us. It's made us stronger, tougher, and more resilient. God has a new purpose for us in all of this. I don't know what it is yet, but I'm glad I get to figure it out with you.

I love you more than you'll ever know. A lifetime doesn't feel like enough time to be your wife. I am going to cherish every second of it even when it's hard.

Love,

Abby

CHAPTER 12

A MOTHER'S HEART

"I prayed for this child, and the Lord has granted me what I asked of him. So now I give him to the Lord. For his whole life he will be given over to the Lord."

~ 1 Samuel 1:27–28a

WHEN I WAS A LITTLE girl, my younger sister, Amanda, and I spent most of our days playing in our backyard. Our entire world was contained within the chain link fence behind our modest house, and we loved every inch of it, despite having to hop and tiptoe around the sharp acorns that regularly stabbed our bare little feet. Whether riding our bikes down the "big" hill, climbing in the wood pile, or pretending to be Mary Lou Retton on our big metal swing set, we were never short on ideas to keep us busy and usually dirty.

My parents spent their weekends in the front yard working on flower beds filled with colorful azaleas and irises, and without fail each spring and summer, our mailbox was surrounded by big yellow and orange marigolds. Our backyard stood in stark contrast to our flower-filled front yard. It was uneven and shade covered, and there were large patches that refused to grow grass. It was far from fancy, but it was the perfect place for two little, adventurous, southern girls to run, jump, dig, and explore.

Grass may have struggled in our backyard, but dandelions flourished. Yellow topped stems speckled the view from our bedroom windows. To Amanda and me, they might as well have been roses. We thought they were beautiful, and we picked them as fast as they could grow. Our mom told us we could use dandelions to tell if someone liked butter, and we believed her. We would pick the golden flowers and hold them under each other's chin to look for a yellow reflection.

When we were done confirming our mutual love of butter, we would bring a small bouquet of flowers into our kitchen. We would climb into a wooden kitchen chair and onto our yellow Formica countertops in order to grab a small paper Dixie cup. We would neatly arrange our dandelions and fill the cup with water before proudly displaying them on the center of the kitchen table. We thought they were magnificent. It wasn't until we were older that we learned most of the world sees dandelions as nothing more than a nuisance, a weed to be treated and destroyed in pursuit of manicured perfection. The voices of others changed our perception and stole the beauty we saw in the weeds.

In much the same way, Wyatt doesn't see the weeds or hardships in his life. He doesn't know his life is difficult. He doesn't understand that everyone doesn't struggle the same way he does. Wyatt doesn't see his wheelchair as a barrier. He sees it as freedom, and he celebrates it. His happiness and joy isn't shaped by outside opinions and beliefs, and he isn't ruled by comparison to society's view of normal or beautiful. He loves the life he lives.

I want to see the world as Wyatt does, void of comparison and worldly expectations. I want to live a life that sees the beauty in the weeds instead of spending all my energy trying to eliminate them. I have seen the beauty in celebrating the hard. I know as a mother I'm supposed to be teaching and encouraging my children to grow into the likeness of Christ. I'm supposed to be a loving, godly example for them. I so badly want to train them up in the way they should go, but I never dreamed my children would be the ones shaping me and teaching me more than I could ever teach them in a thousand lifetimes.

This whole parenting thing is hard. It's a million times harder than I ever thought it would be. Once in Sunday school, I crazily made the statement that I thought God must think a lot of special needs parents to entrust them with such precious children, as if they were magically equipped to handle the challenges of raising a child with special needs. I laugh at myself now for ever thinking such a thing. I had no idea what I was talking about. I am definitely not specially equipped to raise Wyatt, and my value in the eyes of God certainly isn't tied to my parenting ability. God did not give me Wyatt because He thinks more of me than anyone else.

It's easy to lose your identify in the midst of a struggle when you're tired, overwhelmed, and under qualified. Everything feels like too much, and more times than not you feel like a failure at everything. That's been my struggle, especially in a world that expects moms to be everything at all times. I couldn't keep up. We lived off frozen pizza, fish sticks, and sweet tea. I never had time to exercise. I struggled to find more therapy time for Wyatt. My house was never clean enough. I only emptied the kids' school folders on Monday mornings. I didn't throw fancy birthday parties for the kids. Nothing

I did felt like it was good enough, and I didn't feel like I was enough for my family.

I became an emotional wreck set off by the smallest things. More than once, Jason had to dry my tear-covered face after I ruined a blouse or a sweater by getting it caught in the Velcro on Wyatt's braces. I felt like such a big baby sitting on my closet floor crying over a snagged blouse, but it wasn't really the blouse I was crying over. I was crying over my inability to fix my situation. I couldn't make Wyatt better. I couldn't give Jay and Austin all the attention they deserved. It's hard to live a life that you didn't plan, doing something over and over that leaves you feeling totally inadequate and powerless to change it.

I didn't mind the hard so much. Hard is fine with me as long as I know what I'm working toward. It was the powerless part that consumed me. I want to be in control, and I want to know how the story ends. I can't read a fiction book without reading the last chapter first or doing an Internet search to see if my favorite character dies because I don't want to invest my time and energy into a story with an ending I won't like. It's totally insane. I want life to be like a choose-your-own-adventure book where I get to pick the best option, but it doesn't work that way. Sometimes all the options before us hurt. And even though I don't always have the power to change my circumstances, I serve a God who has the power to part seas and bring the dead to life. Jesus died on the cross and rose from the dead, and I am His. Whether I always believe it or not, His power lives in me. When I let that sink into my cluttered mind, it makes me want to shout "Amen" from the back pew. I may not know how the chapters of my life will play out, but I know how the story will end. I've read the last page.

God wins.

I don't why all of this has happened to Wyatt and my family. I don't know why God hasn't reached down to make it all better. I do know that God either ordained it or He allowed it to happen. Either way, I can't change it no matter how hard I cry or how much I beg. I could spend a lifetime being mad at God and demanding answers. The mom in me wants answers. I want to know why Wyatt is paralyzed, but I am a child of God first. Before I am a wife or a mom, I am a daughter of the King of Kings, and I want to live like it even when it hurts. More than anything, I want to trust that God is in control of this messy life I'm living.

I want a faith big enough to let go of all my why questions, and I want to be brave enough to ask how. How can I love God more through my suffering? How can I teach my children more about Him in the midst of heartache? How can I love people more? All the why questions leave me feeling angry and confused, but the how questions give me purpose and a direction. They help me see past the hurt to the blessings in the midst of my storms, and they remind me that God has a purpose for my life.

In chapter 2 of the Gospel of Mark, Jesus heals a paralyzed man. Jesus had traveled to Capernaum. When the people heard Jesus was staying at a home, a large crowd gathered, anxious to hear Jesus speak as word of His miracles had spread. The crowd was so large that it filled the house and spilled out of the door. Four men carried a paralyzed man to the home to see Jesus.

> "Since they could not get him to Jesus because of the crowd,
> they made an opening in the roof above Jesus by digging
> through it and then lowered the mat the man was lying on.
> When Jesus saw their faith, he said to the paralyzed man,
> 'Son, your sins are forgiven'" (Mark 2:4–5).

Teachers of the law had gathered at the home, and when they
heard the words of Jesus, they began thinking to themselves that He
was committing blasphemy. Jesus immediately knew what these men
were thinking in their hearts, and He asked why they were thinking
such things.

> "Which is easier: to say to this paralyzed man, 'Your sins are
> forgiven,' or to say, 'Get up, take your mat and walk'? But
> I want you to know that the Son of Man has authority on
> earth to forgive sins." So he said to the man, "I tell you, get
> up, take your mat and go home." He got up, took his mat
> and walked out in full view of them all (Mark 2:9–12a).

I heard the story countless time growing up, and I was always
astonished at the miracle of the healing. It is the same healing I want
for Wyatt, a whole heart and a whole body. I can only imagine the joy
that must have overtaken this man as he rose off his mat. As I read
this story today, as a mom with a paralyzed son, the Spirit of God
leaves me marveling at something new.

These four men who carried the paralyzed man to Jesus. They are
heroes, and I want to celebrate them. These four men knew the value
of life. They knew love and friendship, and I want to be like them. I
want my kids to surround themselves with friends like them. The
Bible just calls them four men, but I call them four friends because
they loved the paralytic enough to bring him to Jesus. There is no

better friend than the ones who are willing to carry you to the feet of Jesus.

One of these men had to have heard Jesus was close by, and he thought of his friend lying in bed waiting for a miracle. I can imagine him running to the paralyzed man's home to tell him the good news. Healing was near, and the excitement must have been overwhelming. He gathered three friends, and they carried this man down what I can only assume was a rough, dusty road. I wonder what they talked about on the journey. I want to believe they talked about walking home together after a glorious healing had taken place. Their actions revealed a confident heart.

When they got to the home where Jesus was staying, they saw the crowd of people surrounding the house and filling the door ways. The sea of people should have parted. The paralyzed man should have been ushered to the feet of Jesus, but the crowd was too focused on themselves to notice the one with a greater need. These four friends could have given up when God didn't open a door, but these four knew that Jesus was on the other side of the wall. They were so close, and they weren't going to be stopped by a crowded doorway. They were willing to fight to bring their friend to Jesus.

They climbed onto the roof and dug a hole to lower their paralyzed friend to Jesus. I wonder what the crowd outside the home must have thought as they saw this scene unfold before them. Did anyone stop to help them? Did they laugh and point? Did they see the worth in the life of the paralyzed man? The four friends surely did. They were faithful, bold, and persistent. They saw a great need, and they brought their friend to the only One who could fill it.

I want to be that brave! I want to be willing to climb on a rooftop to bring someone to Jesus. Sometimes God calls us to do the hard things, and He doesn't always remove the obstacles before us. Doors don't always fly open before us. I grew up listening to people in the church asking God to open doors for them. Yes, there are times when the doors we are supposed to pass through are standing open, but more often than not, I have found doors to be closed. We have to be willing to fight to accomplish what God has called us to do.

I am reminded of the friends on the roof as I fight for Wyatt. As his parents, Jason and I are the ones who need to bring him to healing. We have been entrusted with his life, and we need to be his fiercest advocates. We need to be willing to set aside our own desires in order to do what is best for our children.

If we truly believe that God has called us to do something, we have to fight to open the door, or we might have to climb on the roof to accomplish the mission before us. We have to trust that God is going to give us the strength. We often have a misconception that because God called us to do something, it should be easy, but the Bible constantly reminds us that this life will be hard.

I have a love-hate relationship with John 16:33: "I have told you these things, so that in me you may have peace. In this world you will have trouble. But take heart! I have overcome the world." I hate the trouble and the certainty of it. It doesn't say might, if, or maybe. It says we *will* have trouble. There is no question. Trouble is going to find us, but thank God the verse doesn't end there. Jesus has overcome! We are not facing our trouble alone.

God is faithful, even when we can't feel Him near us. He is still sovereign even when He is silent. His sovereignty is where I have found my rest. I cannot begin to understand the path Wyatt and my family are on, but I know anything that touches us has passed through the hand of God. He is good, and He will make good from the bad.

I want Wyatt, Jay, and Austin to believe and see the goodness of God in every situation. I don't want them to live a life controlled by the feelings their circumstances create. Feelings are not truth, and feelings will fail them. Truth never will. God is the same in good circumstances and bad. The God standing next to me on the mountain top is the same God who is holding me in the valley.

I want to do more than tell my kids who God is. I want to show them every day and in everything I do. I want to live a life that draws them closer to the One who made them, and my greatest opportunities to do this have come in my weakest moments, when God has made good from the bad. I want to be honest with my kids about my failures and struggles, and I want them to see my great need for a Savior. I don't want to pretend to be superwoman.

I often talk about how God is working through Wyatt's life. I truly believe He is doing amazing things through Wyatt, but I don't want Wyatt to ever mistake those works as a personal relationship. I want to remind Wyatt of his own need for a Savior as he grows. I could work the rest of my life to fight for Wyatt's physical health, but if I neglect his spiritual health, I have failed him completely. If I could have only one wish for each of my children, it would be for them to know Jesus personally, and I pray that my words will always remind them of the one decision that is eternally important. I want Wyatt specifically to know that hardship in this life doesn't create a free pass to heaven.

My Sweet Wyatt,

You are a gift. You are exactly who God intended you to be. If I could line all the little boys up in the world, I would pick you. You are mine, and there is nothing in this world that could make me love you less. You are part of me just like your big brother and sister.

I love your blue eyes and the way they shine when you smile. I love the freckles dotted across the bridge of your nose and the blond curls that sit on the top of your head. I love your precious voice and the way you use the word *actually* like a grown up. You are so smart, and I love to see your mind at work. You are the best puzzle builder I know. You are amazing in every way, and I can't believe that God picked me to be your mom.

You, my boy, are my hero, and I feel so unqualified to guide you through this life. You are everything I wish I could be. You don't know it yet, but you are a warrior. You have fought more in your first four years than most people do in a lifetime, and you smiled through it. You are brave and courageous, and the joy you feel is contagious. You make everyone around you smile.

I wish I was as brave as you. You have more courage and bravery in a single strand of your hair than I have in my whole body. I didn't think I was strong enough to be your mommy. I was so scared when you got sick, and I didn't know what to do. I thought I was going to drown in my own tears. I couldn't stop crying long enough to be brave. I was afraid I was going to lose you, and I couldn't imagine a second of my life without you in it.

You were so little, and Mommies are supposed to make everything better, but I couldn't. I'm so sorry. I'm sorry I couldn't take your pain away. I'm sorry that I couldn't stop it and make it all better. I would give anything to change places with you. I wish it were me instead of you.

I will never stop fighting for you. As long as there is a breath in my body, I will fight to make this life better for you. I will carry you wherever you need to go. I will never stop believing that God can make a way.

I didn't know what your life would look like from a wheelchair. I was scared you would be missing out. I was scared only because I didn't know, but you have shown me. You live life to the fullest, and you've shown me how amazing life can be when you focus on what is possible. You don't waste a single second, and you see the good in every situation.

You are capable of doing anything you put your mind to, brave boy, and I am so thankful to be part of your journey. I have a front row seat to a miracle, and I couldn't be prouder of you. There are so many things I want for your life. My dreams for you haven't changed. They are the same dreams I had for you when you were growing in my womb, and they are the same dreams I have for Jay and Austin. My dreams for you aren't shaped by your disability. It does not define who you are, and don't you ever let anyone make you feel less because you are different.

I know the road before you won't always be filled with confetti and gum drops. There will be hard times. Your heart will get hurt and your soul will be wounded because you are different. People can be stupid, and they are scared of what they don't understand. You will teach them. I can't promise that I can make the hurt go away, but I promise I will always be here to dry your tears. I will always fight for you. I am your biggest fan and your fiercest advocate.

I want you to live a happy and independent life, and I know you will. I want to watch as you spread your joy and grow into the remarkable young man I know you will be. I want to watch as you learn to drive a car. I want to move you into college, and I want to watch you looking down the end of an aisle waiting for your bride. I want to watch you become a father. I want you to dream big and explore all the possibilities this life has to offer, but more than anything else, I want you to know Jesus. He is the only one who can make you whole.

These bodies that you and I live in, they are just temporary homes. Wholeness is about the state of our hearts, not the condition of our bodies. I believe with every ounce of my being that God has big plans for your life. He is already using you, but the choice to follow Jesus will have to be yours alone. Nobody else can decide that for you.

My prayer is that you will see and recognize the goodness of God. I want you to fall in love with Jesus. I pray that you will look past the bad and fight through the hard. I want you to smile even when life hurts and never, ever give up.

I can't even begin to explain how much I love you. My life is better because you are in it, and I can't wait to see the man you become. Conquer the world, my boy. You were made to thrive.

I Love You Forever,

Mommy

CHAPTER 13

CREATED FOR MORE

*I remain confident of this: I will see the goodness of the Lord in
the land of the living.*

~ Psalm 27:13

"MOM, MOM, MOM! I HAVE to tell you a joke!" Wyatt yelled from the back seat of my van. I could hear the excitement in his voice, and I glanced in the rearview mirror to see the expression on his face. His eyes were as big as saucers, and a huge smile filled his face. He was holding his arms straight out before him and opening and closing his hands as fast as he could. The squeezing of his hands had become a tell-tale sign of excitement since he lost the use of his legs and the ability to kick. He couldn't wait one more second for me to answer.

"What do you call an alligator wearing a vest?" he questioned as he clapped his hands in anticipation. "An investigator!" he screamed before I even had a chance to answer. "Isn't that silly, Mommy? An investigator. Do you get it?" His laughter filled the van.

I got it. There was no mistaking it. My little boy was growing up. The baby in the wheelchair is now a blond-haired preschooler who thinks he's ready to take on the world. I blinked, and Wyatt turned four. Four used to seem so far away. It's hard to grasp how quickly time actually slips through our fingers. In some ways, it feels like this battle just began yesterday, but in other ways, I feel like I've aged fifteen years since his diagnosis. As I sort through pictures, I can see years of wear etched across my face. Pain is hard on the mind and body. It leaves a mark on everything it touches. Three years into this battle, there are still moments that take my breath away. Moments that fill me with excitement and joy when a new skill is achieved, and moments that consume my heart with the anguish of affliction when I am reminded of what has been lost.

He bit his toe once. I had just gotten him out of his stander, and I sat him on the couch to wait while I grabbed his medicine. When I walked back to the couch, blood was streaming from his toe. I looked in the socks and shoes I had just removed from his feet. There was no sign of injuries. There was no blood in his sock. I wiped his foot clean, and I still wasn't sure what happened. Finally, Wyatt 'fessed up. He bit his big toe so hard that his teeth went through his toe nail. He never felt it, but every ounce of pain that was spared him was heaped upon my heart.

I don't think I'll ever get used to Wyatt's paralysis. Sometimes as I watch him play, I forget there are things he can't do on his own. He wants to be independent. He rarely uses his wheelchair in the house. He'd rather be on the ground, close to his toys, where he can grab them at will. He army crawls across the floor, dragging his body behind him, determined to get wherever he wants to go. We can track him down by following the trail of lost clothes. Socks and pants inch their way off his body as he crawls oblivious to his skin touching the cold, wood floor. His newest achievement is learning to open the refrigerator. If left unattended, he will remove everything from the bottom shelf and leave it on the kitchen floor. Paralysis has not affected his ability to make a mess. He is a champion mess maker. I have to work on his ability to clean up, or one day his wife will hate me.

As I was finishing up his bath the other day, I held out a towel and asked him to stand up so I could dry him off. I knew what I had done as soon as the words left my lips, but I couldn't take them back. How could I make such a mistake? I was hurrying and careless with my words. Wyatt looked at me with a stare of complete confusion, like I had called him a name he had never heard before.

"Umm, Mom, I can't stand up. Did you think I was Austin?" he asked as he began to laugh.

That was it. He didn't care. It didn't bother him in the least. He laughed at the absurdity of my statement. I felt like my words could have pierced his spirit, but they didn't. He knows who he is. He doesn't have a longing to be anyone else other than who he is. I'm sure one day it will come, but for now, he doesn't ask for healing.

When I put Wyatt to bed each night, I tuck him under his star covered blanket, and we say his prayers together. I guide him in the format, but I let him fill in the blanks. I ask him if there is anything he wants to tell God or ask Him for. He gives me answers, but he has never once said that he wants God to make him better. He's asked God to tell Santa to bring him lots of toys, but he's never asked for healing. So that's not what we pray for together. Healing is still the prayer I pray on my own, but not in front of Wyatt. If I did, he'd tell me he wasn't sick.

He's not sick, and I don't want to forget what a miracle that is. He is truly living this life, not just existing. The first year after Wyatt's paralysis was a survival season. Everything was hard, and we just wanted to make it to the next day, but we've transitioned into a new season. It's been a season of discovery as we navigate the special needs world that we now call home. I cannot begin to tell you how ignorant I was to the special needs community before Wyatt was paralyzed. Everyone in my world was cut from the same cloth as I was, and it was pretty boring.

A lot of my pain from Wyatt's paralysis was caused by my misguided belief that he was going to miss out on so much life. I was wrong. I thought he would be stuck in a chair. He uses a chair, but he is definitely not stuck in it. I had no idea the opportunities that would be available to Wyatt through adaptive sports. He has been able to participate in more by four years of age than most typical children.

He plays baseball through the Miracle League. He's been able to take part in adaptive surfing, wheelchair tennis, hand cycling, and he's even had an opportunity to try out sled hockey. He was amazed at the coldness of the ice beneath his hands when he tried out sled hockey. I couldn't get him to try to push the sled because all he wanted to do was lean over and touch the ice. He hasn't fallen in love with anything, but he's tried everything. That's what is important to me. I want him to grow up knowing that the world is full of possibilities. I want him to grow up seeing the opportunities before him, not the limitations.

On the two-year anniversary of his transverse myelitis attack, Wyatt tried adaptive surfing for the first time. Our family spent the weekend in Myrtle Beach, and Wyatt participated in Wheel to Surf, an adaptive surf clinic for those with disabilities. Adaptive surfers were each assigned to a large team of volunteers who worked to keep them safe in the water while they experienced the thrill of surfing. I was terrified as I watched Wyatt and his team head deeper and deeper into the ocean while he clung to the handles of a long, yellow surfboard.

I didn't realize how far out in the water he would be going. I naively pictured him floating around in knee deep water and riding a few little waves into the shore. I pretty much pictured my childhood days of boogie boarding, but Wyatt was surfing for real. He would not be relegated to the shallow waters. The volunteer team quickly took him out into chest deep water. The white caps of breaking waves danced around them. They were small and unassuming waves, but from where I stood on the beach, they might as well have been waves of epic proportions because I couldn't reach him. A volunteer surfer hopped onto the board with Wyatt and paddled around, waiting for a perfect wave. My heart was pounding in my chest, beating faster every second. I was terrified Wyatt would panic. The mere thought of water in their faces would send Jay and Austin into a tailspin. I was concerned Wyatt would have a meltdown right there in the ocean, but he wasn't rattled. He loved it, water in his face and all.

The first wave pushed his board toward the beach, and the thrill of freedom covered Wyatt's face. There was no fear in him. I cheered as he surfed through the water toward the shore. He was grinning widely as he high-fived me before he was carried back out with his team to catch another wave. I was in awe of my little man and how far he had come.

Just as I began to relax, a large wave knocked Wyatt off the board. My heart sank as I saw Wyatt fall into the water. For a split second, I couldn't see him as he disappeared into the breaking waves, but the volunteer on the board never took his hands off him. They fell from the board and were tossed around a little before the volunteer lifted Wyatt above the water with his hands still firmly under his arms. Wyatt never shed a tear. The smile was still on his face because he trusted the hands holding him.

Two years earlier, I didn't know what his life would look like. I was petrified of the unknown, but standing on the beach, I saw my little boy living a life that was fuller than I could have ever imagined. Though we had been tossed around and often felt as if we were drowning in an ocean of fear, never has God taken His hands off us. He has always been with us. Even when we couldn't feel Him, He was there. God didn't send a miracle in healing, but He sent a miracle to us—a miracle in Himself. We can't choose the events that touch us in this life. We can only choose how we respond to them. If we choose to respond by keeping our eyes on God, we choose to find the good.

We've found good in intentionally making happy memories. Wyatt's medical care has created a lot of opportunities for travel and a lot of time for family bonding inside my van. Worn leather seats and juice-stained carpet are the remnants of adventures taken, time spent together. The odometer has passed 275,000 miles, but it still has more memories than miles. One long autumn weekend, my well-loved van took us to Louisville, KY, for Wyatt to participate in a research study at Frazier Rehab Institute. It turned out to be one of the sweetest times we've had together. Austin still asks me regularly when we're going back to Louisville.

We don't travel often without a purpose or itinerary, but the trip to Louisville almost felt as if we were. The research study took only three to four hours out of our weekend, and then we were free to explore, play, and be normal tourists. We swam in the hotel pool, tried out restaurants, and binge-watched shows on Netflix. I took a nap too. It was glorious! We spent the last day of the trip at Churchill Downs, Home of the Kentucky Derby. We watched the horse races and ate lots of junk food. As it turns out, this was Austin's last eat-anything-you-want hoorah before she was diagnosed with celiac. Austin and I hit the gift shop and took pictures wearing all the fascinators that were way too expensive to ever think about buying. Austin's favorite was a pink one with a big feather.

We stood by the paddocks and watched as the horses paraded to their stalls in preparation for their races. Someone gave Wyatt a pair of jockey goggles to wear. They were just clear plastic with an elastic band, and he easily slipped them on his head himself. He looked like he was getting ready for chemistry class as he rolled around in his chair. He was quite the little scene, and he ended up being brought into the paddock to sit on a horse. I remember watching him sitting on top of that horse with the biggest smile on his face and thinking that moment would never have occurred if Wyatt hadn't been paralyzed.

So much would be different if Wyatt had been healed, but different doesn't mean better. I'm finally beginning to understand that. There is a richness to life that I've never known before. I've lived a hurried life, jumping from one task to another simply to check off boxes on my to-do list. I was productive, but everything I did was void of passion. I was running through life trying to keep up with an imaginary standard I set for myself, and my pursuits never brought me closer to the life I really wanted to live. I wanted a life that brought me closer to the One who created me and a life rooted in the family He gave me.

Life is still busy, full of work, school, doctors' appointments, and therapies, but Wyatt's paralysis has forced me to slow down. There are no quick trips to the store with a child in a wheelchair. Everything I do takes a little planning and thought. I've had to say no to a lot of activities and opportunities, but in saying no, I've said yes to the people I love and the relationships I want to build. Saying no to all the extras allows me the freedom to completely give my whole self to all my yeses. I would rather be completely invested in one thing than to half-heartedly tackle ten.

Wyatt just finished his third summer rehab session in Philadelphia. When I compare where Wyatt is today to that first summer, I am blown away by how much stronger he has become. His arms and shoulders look like a little chiseled statue. He's almost strong enough to do pull-ups in his wheelchair. He already has more muscles in his arms than I ever thought about having. He now uses reciprocating gait orthosis (RGO) to assist with walking over ground. We cheer for the Forrest Gump type braces that brought Jason to tears when Wyatt was diagnosed. The RGOs are orthopedic braces that assist paraplegic patients in walking. They run from the middle of his back all the way down to his feet. The knees and hips both lock to create a standing frame.

The beauty of the RGO braces is a mechanism that accentuates any leg movement Wyatt generates. As Wyatt leans back on his walker to shift his weight, the braces help move his other leg forward into a walk. He still has to have adult assistance and a walker, but he can go so much farther. His therapist, Marci, took him on a field trip to the children's museum. Wyatt was able to alternate between taking steps with a walker in his RGOs and using his wheelchair. It was the first time Wyatt had ever worn the braces in a functional situation outside of therapy.

Wyatt needs close supervision while in the braces because he has no concept of his personal safety. I don't know if it is caused by his lack of physical feeling or simply a product of his young age, but he would fall smackdab on his face if you let him. His quarterly reports from school all state "Wyatt is not safety conscious and flies down ramps." Literally, he throws his arms in the air and pretends like he's flying whenever he goes down a wheelchair ramp.

I definitely don't want Wyatt to get hurt, but I love to see the pure joy and freedom that covers his face when he flies down a ramp. I just try to stand at the bottom to keep him from crashing into anything too terribly hard. It's like any other child climbing to the top of a slide and taking off. There is true exhilaration when you're moving fast enough to feel the wind in your face, and I want Wyatt to be able to feel it as often as he can. I want him to experience as much of the goodness life has to offer as he possibly can.

I still don't like to think about tomorrow. I know Wyatt's fight is going to last a lifetime. Treatment will never end. It will be a way of life. Emotionally, this is as easy as it's ever going to get for him. At four years of age, Wyatt's differences make him cool. His chair is a novelty to his little friends. If he's not sitting in it, they want to climb in and try to wheel themselves around. At fifteen years of age, his differences won't seem so cool. I'm certain that as he grows, he'll begin to ask those why questions, and I pray that God will give me the words to soothe his heart.

Physically, I know there are surgeries on the horizon. So far, we have been lucky. The surgeries have been simple. There has really only been one since the Botox injections. Wyatt had to have his tonsils removed after he developed sleep apnea, but his bladder isn't getting better. He's going to have to have a bladder augmentation in the next few years, and it hurts my heart to think about it. It's a big surgery that can't be undone, but I know we have to do everything we can to keep his kidneys healthy. We've been blessed to avoid any major orthopedic issues. He hasn't developed any major contractures, and he hasn't shown any signs of developing scoliosis. I hope that his TSLO will continue to prevent his spine from curving as he grows.

The medical treatment available to Wyatt is an absolute blessing. Don't think for one second that I ever take it for granted. There are times when I feel guilty because there is a hospital I can drive my son to for care, and there is equipment to make his life easier. None of that happened because of anything I did or anything I deserved. It is simply the grace of God that has us living here with the gift of healthcare. If he had been born on the other side of the world, he would have been left with no options and no hope.

The days are still hard. Our normal rarely looks like anyone else's, but we're okay with that now. We have discovered joy in the life we're living. When everyone else's worst case scenario becomes your life, you have to find a way to move forward, to become brave enough to really live. God didn't create us for an existence of nothingness. We were created for more. To do more. To be more. To love more. More happens when we choose to live beyond our circumstances. More happens when we choose hope instead of despair.

CHAPTER 14

REJOICING IN SUFFERING

*Not only that, but we rejoice in our sufferings, knowing that
suffering produces endurance, and endurance produces character,
and character produces hope, and hope does not put us to shame,
because God's love has been poured into our hearts through the Holy
Spirit who has been given to us.*

~ Romans 5:3–5 (ESV)

I WAS TRYING TO FIND escape from the sun and heat in the shade of a school portable while I waited for Jay's first cross country meet to begin. I tried to coax Wyatt and Austin into the shade with me, but the call of childhood pulled them into the sunshine and had them running and rolling across the grass and uneven terrain behind the school. I stood and watched them play, knowing there was no way for me to keep up with them both as they took off in different directions. I was tired and frustrated from a long day at work, and the task of chasing them seemed like an insurmountable challenge. I was not my best me, and I really just wanted to fuss at them and tell them to stay next to me.

Logic took over, and I let them play. I didn't want to turn my bad day into theirs, and I knew if I let them get tired they might sleep well that night—at least, that was my internal prayer. Wyatt entertained himself near me, and I watched him as he wheeled around looking for a playmate. Before I knew it, he was talking and playing with a boy getting ready to head to soccer practice. Wyatt watched him with amazement as he kicked the ball around dressed in his shin guards and cleats. Wyatt studied him with longing eyes that shouted his heart's desire to play too, and the sweet boy picked up the ball and handed it to Wyatt.

"I can't kick the ball right now," Wyatt said. "But when I grow up, I can kick the ball, but my legs don't work now so I'll just throw the ball."

It was the first time he had uttered those words, and something about them hit me like a ton of bricks. He doesn't think the chair he is in is permanent. When he pictures himself as an adult, he doesn't see the chair. He sees himself standing and running and kicking. I found myself caught off guard by the confident hope he possessed and the giant-sized faith contained in his pint-sized body. He has a hope that doesn't feel sorry for himself today but believes in a better tomorrow. His dreams aren't limited by logic or ability like my own.

I wish I could say that his confidence came from me, but it is all his own. I don't talk about healing or tomorrow very much. I still find it easier to live in the comfort of today and the normal I have grown used to navigating. Tomorrow is still too much. It is the lion I keep caged, hoping I will know how to battle when the cage is opened. I still fight for healing for Wyatt. I search out therapies and look for clinical trials. I won't ever give up on the hope that one day physical healing will come for him, but I had to kick myself when I realized that all my visions of Wyatt's future have him in his chair. When I searched my soul, I realized I found it less painful to envision Wyatt as an adult in his chair instead of risking the heartache of continued unanswered prayers. I wondered if my efforts to protect my own heart were boxing in Wyatt's ability to dream.

That same day, I watched Jay struggle mightily to finish the 3.1-mile cross country course. He is only in the 5th grade, and we hadn't done anything to prepare him for his first cross country season. He didn't yet have the stamina to run the entire course. He was nervous and incredibly worried he'd be laughed at for being slow. He wasn't scared of failure. He was scared of everyone's opinion of his failure. I reassured Jay that no one would be making fun of him, and I would be proud of him no matter what he did. I had only one request. I wanted him to finish the race even if he had to walk. I knew that dropping out of one race would make it easier to drop out of the next. I wanted him to know the value of finishing even if it was hard.

The course he ran was made of three one-mile loops, and when he came around from the first loop, his face was bright red. His sweat-drenched hair was stuck to his forehead. He was exhausted, and the thought of completing two more miles must have seemed like a daunting task. I convinced him that he would feel better if he ran while everyone could see him, and even though he wanted to tell me something different, he ran until he made his way into the woods. Then I waited.

And waited.

I waited long enough that I contemplated going to look for him. Other runners had already finished their race when I saw him appear to come back to me to start his third and final lap. As he came by me, I could see the tears welling up in his eyes, but he kept walking, knowing he would be the last runner to cross the finish line. He was too tired to talk, and he did everything he could to avoid making eye contact. I asked him if he wanted me to walk with him during his last lap. A strong shaking of his head let me know that he wanted his mama to leave him alone.

So I waited again.

It took even longer for him to appear from his final lap, and I worried about how he must have felt knowing that everyone had finished before him. I finally saw him come around the corner from his final lap. His coach met him and encouraged him to run the final leg of the race that traveled across the front of his school to the finish line, and he did. His entire team stood and cheered as he ran as fast as his exhausted body would take him. I wanted to cry at the sight of his entire team cheering for him. His biggest fear was laughter, but instead his effort was met with cheers. I contained my tears, knowing they would certainly embarrass Jay.

More than thirty minutes after the first runners crossed the finish line, Jay finished his first cross country race, and the exhaustion he felt was replaced with a sense of accomplishment that comes only through finishing. The grimace that covered his face was replaced with a smile that was bigger than relief. Wyatt was waiting for Jay and threw his arms ups to congratulate Jay with a brother-sized hug as he shouted, "You won, Jay!"

Jay hadn't come close to finishing first, but he did win that day. He won *his* race because he finished. I didn't realize it when I was a teenager running cross country, but it takes courage to finish last. It takes courage to continue when it hurts and the only reward is completing the race before you. I don't know that I would have been as brave as Jay when I was his age. I probably would have come up with an excuse to quit rather than finish last.

Life is a lot like that. We want to quit and stop when it gets hard. We watch the lives of others, and it seems like the course they are on is so much easier than the one we are traveling. The pain and struggle we are feeling doesn't make sense as we watch others cruise past us with legs and a body that work without effort. We want to stop and quit and question why God hasn't made our path as easy as theirs, and in the midst of the most grueling part of the race when hurts consume us, Gods tells us to rejoice.

To rejoice in our suffering. In our hurt. In our anguish.

How is it possible to rejoice in suffering when every piece of your being wants to curse your situation? I still find myself wrestling with that question when I look at Wyatt. How is a mother supposed to rejoice over her son's broken body? Paralysis is not good. There is not a single part of paralysis that is good or worth celebrating. It is all hard, and I don't think any of it was ever God's plan for His children. Paralysis was never supposed to happen, not to Wyatt, not to anyone, but sin messed up the world. The first bite of the apple shattered everything. Oh, how I wish Eve had known what she was doing when she opened her mouth.

Sin put the hard into this life, and there is nothing that you or I can do to take it away. No amount of good deeds or correct behavior can insulate us from the hurt of this life. Good, bad, saved or lost, the hard will find us all, and it will rip us apart if we let it. In the midst of our brokenness, God calls us to rejoice in Him and not curse the One who could stop it all. It is contrary to every fiber of my human nature. The hard does not make me rejoice. It makes me hurt. Pain, whether physical or emotional, will never be okay with me. I don't rejoice *because* of my suffering, but I can rejoice *in* it. The word *in* is used to show a location, not a reason. I rejoice in my suffering, not because of it. While it is happening, I look for the good. I look to the One who is good, even when I am not. I celebrate the results of the hard. The endurance. The character. The hope.

I wish I could put a pretty ribbon on suffering and tell you that it is easy to rejoice, but I can't. It was hard the day Wyatt was diagnosed, and it was hard this morning when I strapped him into his wheelchair and watched him roll into school. Rejoicing can be hard, but it is healing. Rejoicing points us to the One who is bigger than our hurt. Rejoicing is not a superficial happiness that pretends the hard doesn't hurt.

I don't believe that rejoicing has to look the same for everyone. For me, rejoicing begins with thanksgiving. It begins with an acknowledgment of the blessings before me. Thanksgiving leads me to praise my Maker, and it moves my soul closer to my Father in heaven. It takes my mind off the things in life that I cannot control, and it reminds me of the One who is in control of it all.

For Jason, rejoicing is living a life that is free from anger. It's learning to live life in the darkness of the tunnel instead of waiting for the light at the end of it. It's accepting that God has him in the darkness for a reason, and rejoicing is moving forward with a life of purpose in spite of the darkness.

For Jay, Austin, and Wyatt, rejoicing is breathing in the joy of childhood and exhaling laughter. It is living a life that doesn't see differences, a life of complete and utter trust in the God their parents tell them about. It is believing without question that this life is full of goodness everywhere.

It's not an easy experience to watch your child suffer and to live with affliction as your companion. It aches in the depths of your soul, in places you never knew existed. The world likes to whisper into our ear that time is the healer of our wounds, but time is not a true healer. Time simply creates distance between us and the source of our pain. Time is a Band-Aid that covers our aches from sight. Only Jesus Christ can truly heal the wounds deep inside our hearts. He heals us from the inside out and makes us new. He is the only balm that will ever be able to soothe the aches of sin and suffering.

Wyatt's paralysis has given me a new perspective to view the world and the life I live. The lens through which I see the world is no longer focused on me and my comfort. I used to believe that pain was the worst thing in the world, but Wyatt's paralysis has taught me that there is something much worse than pain. It is the absence of feeling. Pain has a purpose. It is a signal that something is wrong. Wyatt doesn't have that signal in over half of his body, and it makes daily living dangerous for an adventurous little boy who can't feel when he is hurting himself.

As much as I hate to admit it, pain serves a function in our lives. It is not wasted if we address it. It can protect us from destroying ourselves, and it should spur us to correct what ails us. It should cause us to seek out the source of our pain in order to stop it. If our pain is physical, we go to the doctor looking for answers, but sometimes we find it more difficult to see the purpose of the emotional pain that destroys us from the inside out. It's hard to cry out to God when we don't know why we are in the darkness. It's hard to accept that God has allowed pain in any form to find us. It can cause us to doubt His goodness and sovereignty.

I don't know your struggle. I don't know if you are in the middle of a raging storm being tossed by ferocious waves or wading in calm, crystal waters, but I do know that Christ longs to be near you in either place. He is the same on the top of the mountain and in the valley. If you are a child of the Risen King and God hasn't pulled you from the darkness, He has a purpose for it. You have not been forgotten, my friend. Call out to God and ask Him to show you His goodness and rejoice in the fact that our hope extends beyond the life we are living. Even if God doesn't bring the healing we crave in this life, eternity beckons. This life is not the end.

If you haven't met Jesus yet, He is calling you in the middle of the darkness. He is calling you in the middle of the calm waters. He is calling you wherever you are to live a life that is filled with the hope that only He can provide. Open your ears. Open your heart. He is calling. He is calling you through a little boy in an orange chair.

It's hard to reconcile suffering with the goodness of God. It is a battle that I will never completely understand. There are still days when I get angry, confused, and bitter, but I choose to focus on what I know to be true. God loves me anyway. And He loves you. And that is where my hope will rest, not in medicine or healing, but in the unfailing love of a Savior. Who sees me. Who knows me. And who loves me in spite of it all. Anyway.

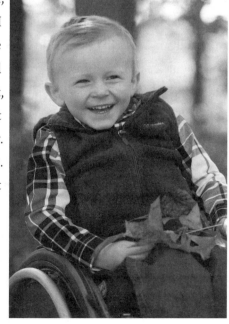

ACKNOWLEDGMENTS

Books are hard to write, harder than I ever imagined, but this section has caused me to fret more than anything else. It's because I am *horrible* at thank yous. It is one of my greatest character flaws. I know it, and I am working diligently to correct it. If you did something kind for me or my family, you probably never received a thank you card. I sincerely apologize. My lack of acknowledgment is in no way reflective of the appreciation that pumps through my heart. If Jason could change only one thing about me, I am convinced it would be this.

I could fill a million pages with fancy words, and it wouldn't come close to enough to thank all the people who have loved my family, who have poured into us, and who have prayed without ceasing. Like in Exodus when Aaron and Hur held the arms of Moses in the air when he was too weak to do it on his own, you have carried us when we didn't have the strength to move forward. Friends, family, doctors, nurses, therapists, social workers, and complete strangers have supported us from the very beginning. We have been blessed beyond measure by so many who have fallen in love with Wyatt.

To Jason: I am so glad I get to call you mine. There is no one I would rather navigate this wild life with than you. Thank you for encouraging me to chase my crazy dreams and letting me share our family's story. Your advice and opinions have been invaluable as I have struggled to put words on paper. I hope this little endeavor of mine makes you proud.

To Jay, Austin, and Wyatt: I love you three to pieces. I want to push pause on our lives and keep you this age a little longer. Y'all are so much fun! Thank you for letting mommy write. I know you grew tired of seeing me sit in front of a computer and of eating cereal and sandwiches for dinner. Thank you for being patient with me. So much of this book was written so you will never forget the battles you have won. I gave birth to my heroes.

To Mom and Dad: Thank you for giving so much of yourselves to us. We could not have survived without your constant support. You have always been there for us whether it was here, Baltimore, or Philadelphia. Thank you for always showing up and letting Jason and me rest whenever we needed it. Thank you for loving us abundantly and for teaching me to never give up. I love you both so much.

To Walter: You have always been at work behind the scenes in our lives. Thank you for keeping our little empire running so Jason and I could forget about everything and focus on Wyatt. I'm so glad you didn't choose a "normal" life all those years ago. If you had, we would not have been able to stay by Wyatt's side day and night. Thank you for sacrificing some of your golden years to help us. I know you'd much rather spend your days fishing and bush hogging.

To Gayla: It breaks my heart that you cannot remember a moment of our story, but I promise your grandchildren will never forget a moment of yours. Thank you for raising such amazing children. They are so much of you.

To Amanda and Kevin, Robin and Ed, and Mandie and David: Thank you for dropping everything in your own lives to care for our kids. We never once worried about who would take care of Jay and Austin when we left with Wyatt. Thank you for loving our children like your own. We're blessed to have the most amazing sisters and brothers-in-law.

To Uncle Shorty: Thank you for being our biggest prayer warrior.

To our Philadelphia family: Getting to be part of your lives again has been an unexpected blessing of Wyatt's condition. Thank you for stopping everything to pick us up at the airport, visit us at the hospital, and join us for dinner.

To Tim Lowry and Ambassador International: Thank you for believing our story was worth telling and taking a chance on a writer who didn't even know what a book proposal was supposed to look like.

And finally to Jesus, the one who paid my debt: This thank you is the hardest because no words will ever be adequate to thank a God who knows all of my flaws and loves me anyway. You are the King of Kings, yet you know my name. May I always be in awe of that fact. Since I know my words will never be enough, I pray my life will be a picture of my thanksgiving to You. May the life I live honor You in every way. I long for the day I hear You say, "Well done, my good and faithful servant."

For more information about

Abby Banks

and

Love Him Anyway
please visit:

www.fightlikewyatt.com
abbybanks@fightlikewyatt.com
@fightlikewyatt
Instagram: @fightlikewyatt, @abbywbanks
www.facebook.com/wyattsfightagainsttm

For more information about
AMBASSADOR INTERNATIONAL
please visit:

www.ambassador-international.com
@AmbassadorIntl
www.facebook.com/AmbassadorIntl